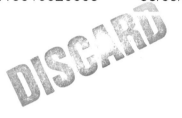

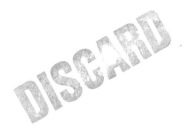

the Quiet Hero

The Quiet Hero

A Life of Ryan White

by Nelson Price

INDIANA HISTORICAL SOCIETY PRESS | INDIANAPOLIS 2015

© 2015 Indiana Historical Society Press

This book is a publication of the
Indiana Historical Society Press
Eugene and Marilyn Glick Indiana History Center
450 West Ohio Street
Indianapolis, Indiana 45202-3269 USA
www.indianahistory.org
Telephone orders 1-800-447-1830
Fax orders 1-317-234-0562
Online orders @ http://shop.indianahistory.org

Library of Congress Cataloging-in-Publication Data

Price, Nelson.
The quiet hero : a life of Ryan White / Nelson Price.
    pages cm
Includes index.
ISBN 978-0-87195-307-0 (cloth : alkaline paper)
1. White, Ryan. 2. White, Ryan—Health. 3. AIDS (Disease)—Patients—Indiana—Biography.
4. Heroes—Indiana—Biography. 5. AIDS (Disease) in children—Social aspects. 6. AIDS
(Disease)—Patients—Education. I. Title.
RJ387.A25P75 2013
618.92'97920092—dc23
[B]
                        2012044761

The paper in this publication meets the minimum requirements of American National Standard
for Information Sciences—Permanence of Paper for Printed Library Materials,
ANSI Z39. 48–1984 ∞

This book is dedicated
to all young people
confronted by challenges.

Contents

"My name is Ryan White. I am sixteen years old. I have hemophilia, and I have AIDS."

Preface

I met Ryan White, soon after the initial stream of reports about a fourteen-year-old boy with Acquired Immune Deficiency Syndrome who was crusading to attend school, in the bedroom of his one-story, ranch home in Kokomo, Indiana. The reports in early 1986 had intrigued me as a young, Indianapolis-based journalist because they touched both on my previous newsbeat as well as on my new, feature-oriented area of focus. At the *Indianapolis News*, the sister newspaper of the *Indianapolis Star*, I had started out as the education beat reporter. Now, I was transitioning to a position as a feature writer/columnist with a focus on writing profiles of Hoosier newsmakers.

Scrawny, frail Ryan seemed like an intriguing, and unlikely, newsmaker. Here was a kid in a bedroom furnished with GI Joes, a stash of Spider Man comic books, and a waterbed covered by a camouflaged-patterned spread that was just becoming wildly popular. I was full of questions that I sensed my readers shared. Top among them: Why was Ryan, while he struggled with a disorder then regarded as a death sentence and which created widespread panic, determined to attend classes at Western Middle School in nearby Russiaville, Indiana?

My initial profile of Ryan and his steadfast mother, Jeanne, attempted to illuminate the people and issues in the explosive controversy that eventually made Ryan a nationally known figure. For the next several years, I covered various aspects of Ryan and his family's saga, even as the *News* merged with the *Star*.

On April 8, 1990, a chilly, spring morning, Ryan died. I was among the throng of media and other visitors—ranging from neighbors, Hamilton Heights High School classmates, and other mourners to camera-toting gawkers—assembled on the lawn of the Whites' house in Cicero, Indiana, where they had moved. Two years later, I reported about Jeanne's marriage to one of those Cicero neighbors, a mechanic and divorced father named Roy Ginder. I never really lost touch with Jeanne; eventually, I included Ryan and his mother in my first book, *Indiana Legends: Famous Hoosiers from Johnny Appleseed to David Letterman*.

In what seemed like a flash, it was 2010. I had left the newspaper to focus on my books and on a Hoosier history radio show that I host. Ryan had been gone for twenty years, and Ray E. Boomhower, editor of *Traces of Indiana and Midwestern History*, was asking me to write a retrospective article about Ryan for the quarterly magazine published by the Indiana Historical Society.

This book evolved from that. I have reinterviewed many of the major figures in Ryan's life, and, in the case of several others, interviewed them for the first time. They include Doctor Martin Kleiman, the infectious disease specialist at Riley Hospital for Children in Indianapolis who became Ryan's personal physician; Heather McNew Stephenson, the classmate Ryan had planned to escort to the prom; and Doctor Jill Stewart Waibel, whose journey has taken her from student body president at Hamilton Heights to a career as a surgeon.

I'm grateful to them, as well as to Jeanne White-Ginder, who patiently answered my waves of fresh questions during several reinterviews; Ron Colby, former principal of Western Middle School; Dan Carter, a retired teacher who headed the Western School District's board during the controversy; Doctor Woodrow Myers, the former commissioner for the Indiana Department of Health; and many others whose insights helped shape this book. All of them answered my questions fully and openly. In addition, Jeanne provided most of the images of Ryan used in this book.

When I was about halfway through with the legwork, I was alerted about a project under way in Howard County, Indiana. Allen Safianow, professor emeritus of history at Indiana University at Kokomo and a guest on my *Hoosier History Live!* radio show on WICR-FM, mentioned he and other members of the Howard County Historical Society were undertaking a community-wide oral history project about the Ryan White school controversy. Insights the Howard County volunteers amassed have helped strengthen this book, so I'm appropriately grateful. And, with Ryan obviously unavailable for further interviews, *Ryan White: My Own Story*, his autobiography cowritten with Ann Marie Cunningham and published posthumously, was valuable in capturing his perspective.

Finally, I'm grateful the Indiana Historical Society Press has recognized the importance of telling Ryan's story to new generations—and to tell it in an inclusive way, with the voices of a range of residents from communities who lived through it. In many ways, Ryan's story is about communities. On the other hand, it's also about the power of one.

"I don't want to be treated worse than other kids, but I don't want to be treated better either. I just want to be the same."

1

During the 1980s, a mysterious disorder created panic across the United States, as well as in other parts of the world. People were dying from Acquired Immune Deficiency Syndrome, which quickly became commonly known as AIDS. Victims ranged from movie stars and other celebrities to newborn infants, children, and residents of small towns. Many victims were drug addicts, hospital patients who had received blood transfusions, and homosexuals.

In addition to sparking alarm—and partially because of the terrified public reaction—the AIDS epidemic spawned confusion, misunderstanding, and intolerance. That fact that people did not know for sure how this previously unknown disorder was being transmitted created almost as many controversies and as much strife as the disorder itself.

At the epicenter of the national panic was a scrawny, sandy-haired, fourteen-year-old boy from Kokomo, Indiana—Ryan White. Ryan lived near the outskirts of town in a modest, ranch-style house with his mother, Jeanne, and younger sister, Andrea. He liked X-Men comic books, Mexican food at Chi Chi's Restaurants, pop music, blue jeans with a sharp crease, and professional basketball stars. (Having struggled with health issues from birth, Ryan always was short for his age, partially explaining his admiration for towering athletes.) Ryan was diagnosed with AIDS just before the Christmas holiday season of 1984, shortly after his thirteenth birthday on December 6.

Probably more than anything else, Ryan wanted to be a normal midwestern kid. That included going to school with his friends, who attended Western Middle School in Russiaville, which borders the southwestern edge of Kokomo in Howard County. His crusade to attend school—in spite of pockets of intense opposition and open hostility in his community—eventually made the pale, straight-speaking boy with a raspy Hoosier twang famous.

Hailed as a "kid pioneer," Ryan testified before a committee of U.S. Congress and cabinet members in Washington, D.C. He was named a "Person of the Week" by ABC News, featured several times on the cover of *People* magazine, and befriended by celebrities such as rock stars Elton John and Michael Jackson. A television-movie about his life, *The Ryan White Story*, was broadcast in 1989. He created such an impact that presidents from George H. W. Bush to Barack Obama have, in Ryan's name, signed legislation to help thousands of Americans with AIDS.

"I Know I'm Somebody 'Cuz God Don't Make No Junk" was the message on a bumper sticker that Ryan affixed to his bedroom wall. The bumper sticker expressed his attitude about self-worth, which profoundly influenced people ranging from international celebrities to residents of small towns. Even more than twenty years after Ryan died at age eighteen on April 8, 1990, and at a glittering event in New York City, far from the suburban midwestern subdivisions where Ryan had lived, Elton John told a group of powerful Americans that the boy from Indiana had changed his life and taught the nation tolerance.

"It took the death of Ryan White before this country did anything about AIDS," said John, who then performed his mournful song about early death, "Candle in the Wind," in Ryan's memory. Similarly, Jackson, a native of Gary, Indiana, recorded a ballad, "Gone Too Soon," in 1991 and dedicated it to Ryan.

In *Love is the Cure,* John's memoir about the AIDS epidemic, he credited Ryan, and the teenager's fortitude when confronted with intense hostility and with a fatal disorder, with saving the pop superstar's life. "I'm here today because of Ryan," John wrote, revealing he was self-absorbed, addicted to drugs, and indulging in a fast-paced lifestyle when he met Ryan. "It took Ryan's death to wake me up, to transform my life . . . I loved that he didn't have an ounce of quit in his heart. . . . In the end, Ryan wound up reaching far more than those in Kokomo, Indiana. He reached the entire nation."

At Riley Hospital for Children in Indianapolis, John had joined Jeanne and other family members and friends in a bedside vigil while Ryan was dying. After that, he performed during Ryan's funeral at Second Presbyterian Church in the Hoosier capital. Selected because the massive church has one of the largest sanctuaries in the state, Second Presbyterian was packed with 1,500 mourners ranging from then-First Lady Barbara Bush and Jackson to Ryan's classmates at Hamilton Heights High School in Cicero, where he had lived for the final three years of his life. During the memorial service, which was broadcast live on CNN, John performed a diverse selection of music that brought many to tears. On the orders of Governor Evan Bayh, Indiana's flag was flown at half-mast across the state.

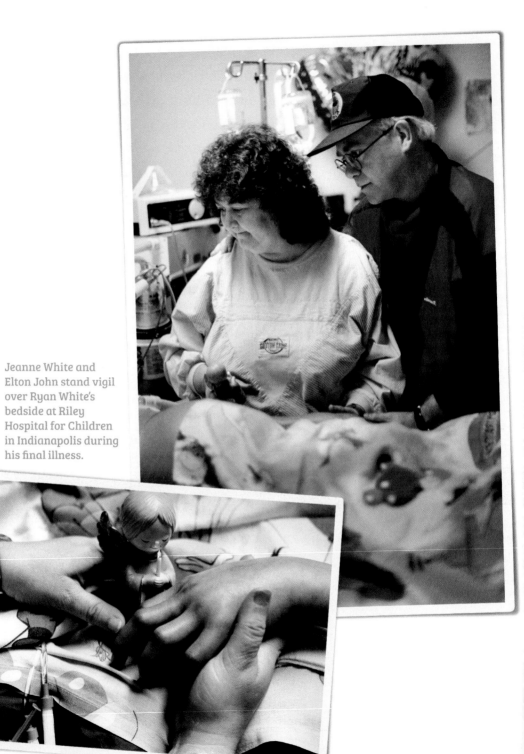

Jeanne White and Elton John stand vigil over Ryan White's bedside at Riley Hospital for Children in Indianapolis during his final illness.

At the Children's Museum of Indianapolis a permanent exhibition, *The Power of Children: Making a Difference*, celebrates the lives of three young people who confronted overwhelming odds and became courageous figures to millions. In addition to Ryan, whose bedroom furniture from Cicero is displayed, the exhibition salutes Anne Frank of the Netherlands, who was thirteen when she began hiding from the Nazis—and also started describing her experiences in a diary—during the Holocaust in World War II. The exhibition

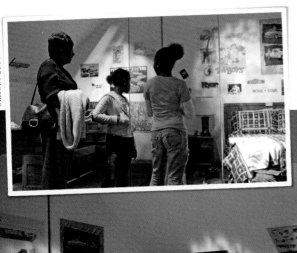

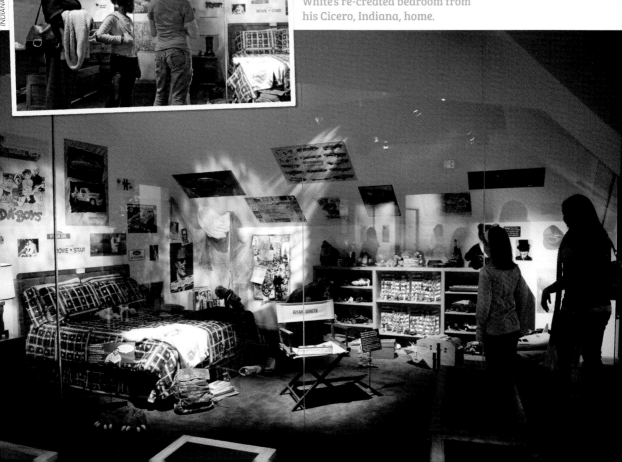

Visitors to the Children's Museum of Indianapolis examine Ryan White's re-created bedroom from his Cicero, Indiana, home.

also honors Ruby Bridges, an African American girl who, as a first grader, integrated schools in the Deep South by walking through angry mobs during the early 1960s.

"I just want to tell everyone something—please don't hate us," Ryan said in 1987, referring to AIDS patients. He made the spontaneous remark, which was typical of his blunt, disarming approach, at Hamilton Heights High School during a press conference after Indiana governor Robert Orr honored the teenager with the state's Sagamore of the Wabash award. Dozens of his classmates at Hamilton Heights also received an award, a newly created "Spirit of the Heartland" honor, for embracing and supporting Ryan and his family after they moved from Kokomo to Cicero in Hamilton County.

"Here was this teenager carrying this huge burden, but he made it seem effortless," said Doctor Jill Stewart Waibel, a surgeon in Florida. As student body president in the late 1980s at Hamilton Heights, Waibel became one of Ryan's friends and joined him in testifying before congressional leaders. "He didn't enjoy the media, and I kept telling him, 'Ryan, you don't *have* to do all of these speeches and appearances.' He said, 'Yes, I do. I don't want others to suffer,'" she said.

"Ryan changed my life, and he enlightened so many, many people," said Heather Stephenson, a special education teacher in Carmel, Indiana. As a vivacious, dark-haired teenager named Heather McNew, she was Ryan's biology lab partner at Hamilton Heights and quickly became his best friend. Together they visited Jackson's Neverland Ranch, spent endless hours cruising around a popular teen hangout in Ryan's red Mustang (the sporty car, Ryan's prized possession during his final years, was a gift from Jackson), and worked on the yearbook staff.

Heather and Ryan planned to attend the school's prom together in late April 1990. Ryan even expressed a preference about the dress he wanted Heather to wear on their big night. "It should be emerald green—that's your color," he told her.

Instead of preparing for the prom, Heather found herself joining Jeanne, Andrea, John, Ryan's physician Doctor Martin Kleiman, and a tight-knit group of other caregivers, friends, and relatives in the bedside vigil at Riley Hospital. Ryan was in critical condition for several days and slipped into a coma before his death, which made national news.

Former president Ronald Reagan, who had met Ryan near the end of his life, praised the Hoosier teenager in a tribute. "We owe it to Ryan to open our hearts and our minds to those with AIDS," Reagan wrote in the tribute, which was published on the day of the funeral. "We owe it to Ryan to be compassionate, caring, and tolerant toward those with AIDS, their families, and friends. It's the disease that's frightening, not the people who have it."

Almost every aspect of the disorder had terrified the public since the first reports about what became known as AIDS were published in 1981. Throughout the 1980s, a diagnosis of AIDS was akin to a death sentence; the disorder ravages people's immune systems, leaving them vulnerable to an array of powerful infections and viruses such as pneumonia. Fatalities were increasing rapidly every year. In 1983 Americans who died of AIDS-related causes totaled about 1,290, which accounted for more than half of the people diagnosed with it. In 1985 the number of AIDS-related deaths in the United States had more than quadrupled to 5,636.

In many ways, Ryan humanized AIDS patients to millions of Americans because he came across on national televsion as a typical midwestern teenager, albeit a quick-thinking one with steely resolve. "Ryan always knew what he wanted, which was to seek normalcy," recalled Doctor Woodrow Myers, the Indiana health commissioner in the 1980s who, like Ryan, became a lightning rod for criticism during the controversy. "He wanted to go on dates, he wanted to have a car, he wanted to be as normal as possible— which, of course, made him so effective once he found himself in the national spotlight."

Ryan often disliked the media focus on him, particularly if the attention felt intrusive at school or at home. Sometimes he lingered in his bedroom after instructing his mother how to deal with reporters waiting in the living room. When speaking before large audiences of people, Ryan grew comfortable once he realized he was making an impact. He eventually told his life story and answered intensely personal questions about his health and life expectancy

Ryan relaxes with a comic book and his family's pet cat, Chi Chi.

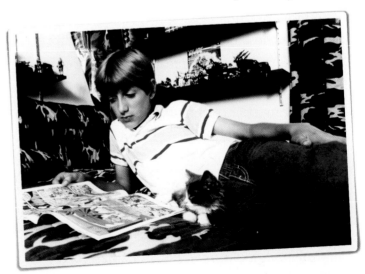

at convention halls filed with thousands of people of all ages. He always preferred speaking to children and teenagers, though. "Kids listen," he explained.

For years before the AIDS diagnosis, and for several months after it, Ryan had not been the focus of much attention at all. Not

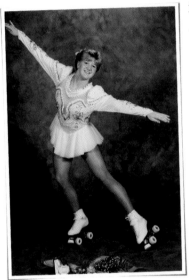

in his neighborhood in Kokomo, and not even within his small family. His sister Andrea, who was two years younger, exuded robust health and enjoyed spectacular success as a roller skater. As a twelve-year-old she won a state championship for her age group, placed third in a Midwest regional, and qualified for a national tournament.

Unfazed by hard falls, scrapes, and tumbles that would have devastated her frail brother (Ryan suffered from severe hemophilia, a disorder that prevented his blood from clotting and meant even minor injuries could be life threatening), Andrea excelled in freestyle roller skating events. Her repertoire included a dazzling, seven-jump combination that featured a double flip—a real crowd pleaser.

Ryan, on the other hand, always had to be extra careful when playing sports or roughhousing with friends and his pets. If he hurt himself, he could bleed to death. Sometimes, he endured intense pain and had to be rushed to the hospital with what the Whites called a "bleed" even if he rolled over in bed on one of his toy matchbox cars. Hemophilia, which is more common in boys and men than in girls and women, affects about 20,000 Americans. Although almost all of them are born with the disorder, it can go undetected for years until an injury results in uncontrolled bleeding.

Because of his hemophilia, Ryan had to take special medicine, including a liquid agent known as Factor VIII that helped his blood to clot. Jeanne injected the Factor VIII in Ryan with a small needle. She stored eight to twelve boxes of Factor VIII in the family's refrigerator, and Ryan received the injections twice a week.

Eventually, medical experts and the White family concluded that contaminated Factor VIII medicine had transmitted the AIDS virus to Ryan. During the early 1980s, before a full understanding of the ways AIDS and other infectious diseases could be transmitted, hospitals and health-care facilities did not screen blood and related products, such as Factor VIII, in the careful ways they have done subsequently.

Ryan's severe hemophilia caused countless hospitalizations in the years after his birth in 1971. As a result, early in his life Ryan became deeply knowledgeable and insightful about medical issues, qualities he eventually used in a way that may have saved his grandfather's life.

"He was thirteen years of age when I met him, but it was like talking to an adult," Kleiman recalled years later. "In fact, in many ways Ryan was more 'adult' than most people ever become in their lives."

But the chronic illnesses also meant that, rather than join Andrea in roller skating and other sports, he had to sit among the spectators. Ryan was taken by his mom to so many of his sister's tournaments across Indiana that he began to shun them.

"I can't say as I blame him," Jeanne said at one point. Yet she did not have many choices about taking him with her. When Ryan and Andrea were about six and four years old, Jeanne divorced Ryan's father, Wayne White. He did not speak in public and never assumed a role in the explosive debates surrounding his son's school attendance. In *Ryan White: My Own* Story, an autobiography published after his death, Ryan and coauthor Ann Marie Cunningham noted that he and Andrea "didn't see Dad much at all" after their parents' divorce. Jeanne did credit her ex-husband,

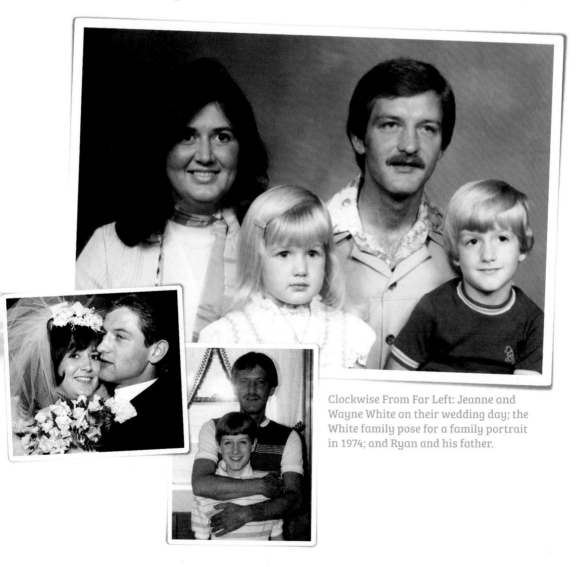

Clockwise From Far Left: Jeanne and Wayne White on their wedding day; the White family pose for a family portrait in 1974; and Ryan and his father.

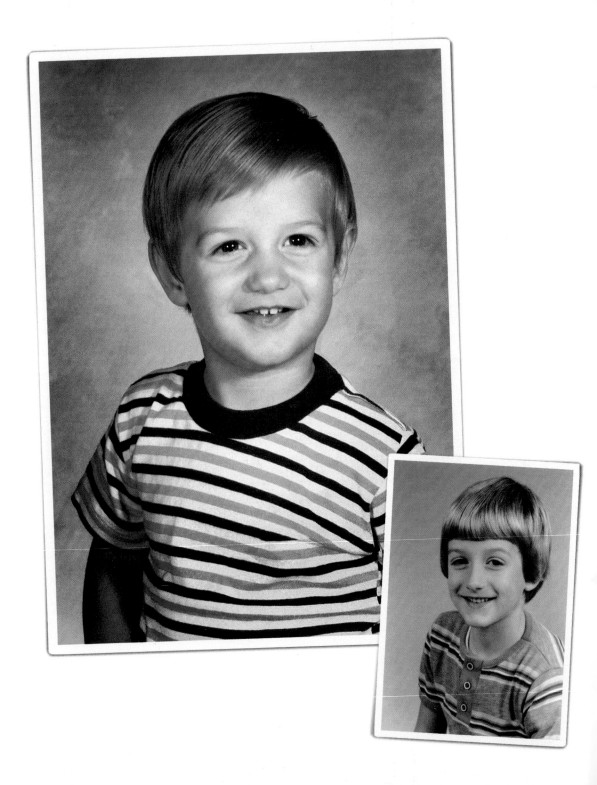

though, with regularly maintaining his child-support payments.

The money was crucial because Jeanne's pay from her job at a factory in Kokomo was stretched by ever-mounting bills. She began work at Delco Electronics Corporation shortly after graduating from Kokomo High School in 1965. The factory produced automobile engines and electronics, including car radios. Her job was repetitive and occasionally stressful. But a small group of her Delco coworkers provided desperately needed assistance in a nonfinancial way: They offered emotional support when Jeanne felt besieged.

Her coworkers, along with Jeanne's parents and other relatives, became cherished stalwarts in Howard County when, because of Ryan's AIDS diagnosis and his determination to attend school, a controversy erupted. It made national headlines and became, as Jeanne put it, a "nightmare."

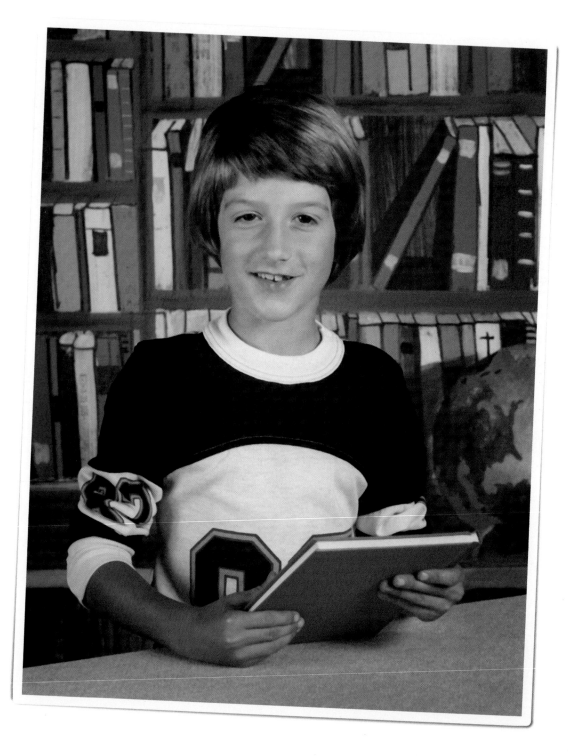

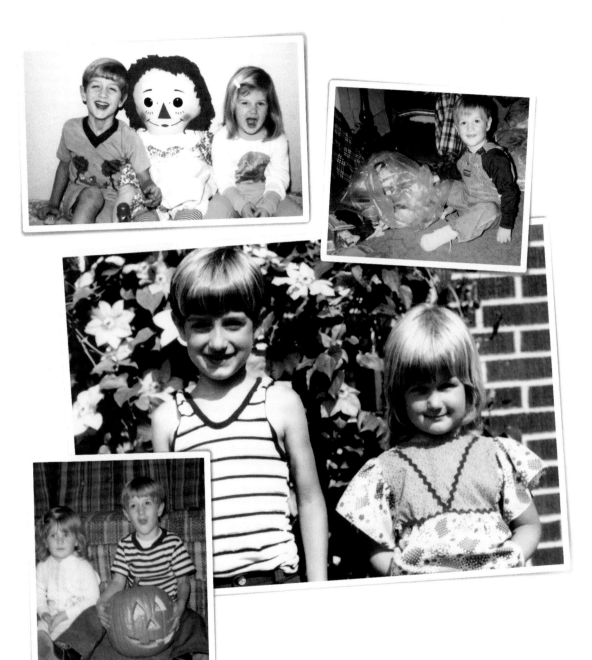

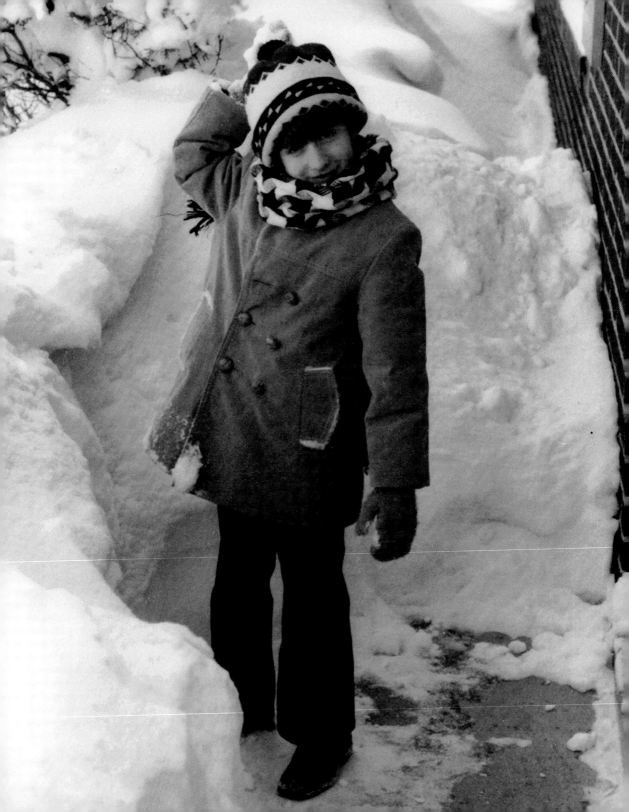

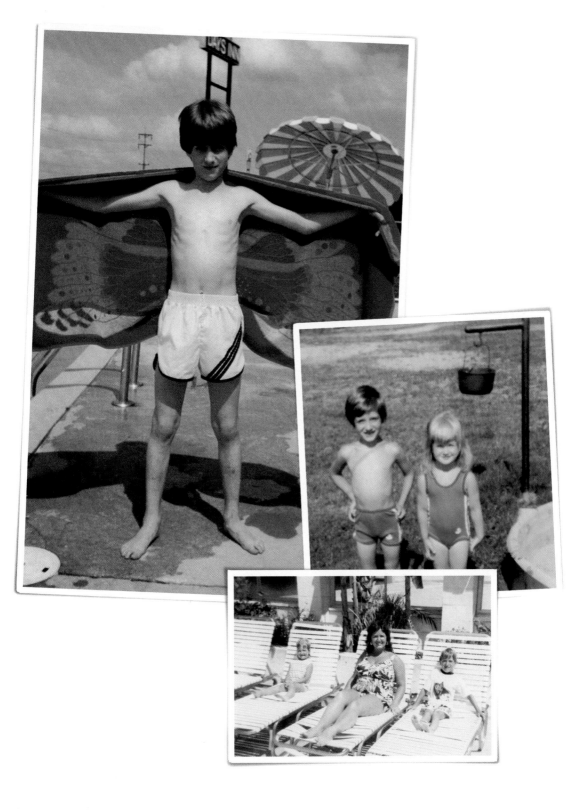

"All I ever wanted to do was be one of the kids, because that's what counts in high school. That and graduating."

2

"You know, Ryan's been seen spitting on grapes in grocery stores." Some residents of the Kokomo area whispered that and other far-fetched rumors to their neighbors and repeated them to out-of-town television and newspaper reporters. One of Ryan White's best friends, when both were barely fourteen, was repeatedly called a "fag" because he stuck by his buddy with AIDS.

A group of parents fought Ryan's crusade to attend Western Middle School with a lawsuit. When they exhausted their appeals, some parents pulled their children and set up a private school so their sons and daughters would not have to be in class with him. Even some teachers asked not to have him assigned to their classrooms.

Callers to radio stations in Howard County expressed such hostility and even rage that Ryan's grandmother, Gloria Hale, often was reduced to tears, and, eventually, to phoning in herself to defend her family.

Reporters for *Newsweek* and other national publications asked Jeanne White if she and her daughter Andrea shared toothbrushes with Ryan. Their readers were curious about such matters, the journalists explained.

Even three years later, after the Whites had moved to Cicero following intensive local education campaigns about AIDS, fifteen-year-old Heather McNew lost a babysitting job when a mother found out she had become Ryan's best friend at his new school. "I just can't take a chance on having you around my children," she told Heather. Tucked inside her locker at Hamilton Heights High School, Heather occasionally would discover vicious, anonymous notes from classmates about her friendship with Ryan.

On the other side of the controversy, an anonymous caller threatened Dan Carter, president of the Western School District's board in Howard County. The caller denounced Carter and other school officials for "tormenting" Ryan after board members took what they felt was a principled decision to uphold a provision in Indiana law prohibiting admitting a student with an infectious disease to school when the local health official advised against it, which was the initial situation with Ryan's request.

At one point, the media coverage at Western Middle School was so intense and intrusive that some newspaper and televsion news teams arrived in helicopters that landed near elementary school playgrounds. "The little kids were terrified," recalled Ron Colby, principal of Western Middle School. "They thought it was an alien invasion."

Is it any wonder the controversy about Ryan's crusade to attend school seemed like a "nightmare" to so many of the people involved?

"Personally, I would rather have given it up a long time ago," Jeanne conceded in early 1986. Seated in the living room of her home in Kokomo while Ryan rearranged his GI Joes in his bedroom, Jeanne confided her preferences during the heat of the controversy.

Immediately backing off or abandoning the crusade for Ryan to attend school after opposition exploded, she said, "would have been a lot easier on me, and a lot easier on the rest of the family. . . . But this is what Ryan wants to do, and I want what he wants." Underscoring the point, she emphasized that any parent of children stricken with a fatal disorder would fight ferociously to ensure they could spend their days the way they desired.

Although Ryan's crusade to attend school received by far the most national publicity and he came to symbolize all young people with AIDS, other families and school districts across the country in the 1980s struggled with similar issues as panic and uncertainty spread. In Florida, six-year-old triplets with the AIDS virus were barred from school in 1985. Eventually, Dade County officials decided to have a volunteer teacher educate the triplets in a separate classroom at a building that was mostly empty. "AIDS is two epidemics," Doctor Jeffrey J. Sacks, the state epidemiologist in Florida, told the *New York Times*. "It's an epidemic of disease and death, but it's also been an epidemic of fear."

None of the fury and frenzy surrounding Ryan could have been predicted when he was born in Methodist Hospital in Indianapolis on December 6, 1971. He confronted major medical challenges almost from the beginning, though. At first, he looked deceptively healthy. Even as a newborn baby, Ryan had thick hair. He also had big feet.

But when surgeons at Methodist performed a minor medical procedure on Ryan, he bled so continuously that doctors felt compelled to run a series of tests. Then they told Jeanne they needed to talk to her. They informed her that her newborn son was a severe hemophiliac and had less than 1 percent clotting factor in his blood.

"You will have to be very cautious," they advised her. Ryan could never play contact sports. He probably could not survive a car accident because Ryan would lose blood faster than it could be pumped into him. The doctors kept emphasizing how fragile Ryan's health would be for his entire life. "I thought, 'Please God, no, not this,'" Jeanne recalled in the mid-1980s, by which point far more serious health challenges were confronting Ryan.

Almost from the beginning, though, Ryan was determined to be like other kids. When he was three years old, he and a playmate in Kokomo could not resist using Jeanne and Wayne's bed as a trampoline. They climbed on top of the bed and began bouncing. Ryan eventually lost his balance and tumbled off, banging his elbow against an electric heater as he fell. Unable to move his arm, he was rushed to the hospital, where doctors detected breaks in three places. After being hospitalized for several days, Ryan was released, with his arm in a sling.

"The worst part was the way I stood out at day care," he recalled in his autobiography. "Everyone asked me, 'What happened?' When I said, 'I got a bleed,' they asked, 'What's that?' . . . I had to give a long explanation. It was very boring, talking about hemophilia over and over, and I sincerely wished I could be invisible until my arm healed."

Yet, Ryan concluded there were positive aspects about the hospitalization, which was followed by many others. They included an emergency trip after he rolled over in bed on one of the half dozen matchbox cars that he liked to sleep with. So what were the positive aspects of the hospitalizations? From a young age, Ryan figured out, as he put it, "how to handle pain."

Ryan explained it this way in his autobiography: "It's real easy to let the pain take over because there's not much else to think about. You need as much distraction as possible. Once I started practicing about not thinking about pain, I got to be fairly good at picking up a magazine until that didn't work anymore, then trying the TV, and after that setting up my GI Joes. The trick is to have a lot of different things to do, because each one can work for only so long."

Ryan also developed a stubborn streak. If he wanted to do something, he would find a way to make it happen, a pattern that continued after he was diagnosed with AIDS. An example was his desire to have pets. Because AIDS attacks people's immune systems and makes them vulnerable to all kinds of infections and viruses, medical specialists initially worried about the risk of infections from household animals. They recommended the White family not own any pets. Ryan balked. He told his mother: "It's my life, and I want a pup. I want a pup that likes no one but me."

He was so insistent about having a dog that Jeanne eventually caved in, as she did with many of his requests. The Whites adopted a mixed-breed mutt named Wally. Jeanne, Ryan, and Andrea also got a cat, Chi Chi.

From the beginning, Ryan and Andrea developed a close bond. When Andrea, who was born in 1973, was an infant, her older brother enjoyed rubbing rice pudding in her hair. Andrea would react by giggling. As she grew, Andrea increasingly became, to use her mother's word, a "tomboy." Her enthusiasm for sports, particularly roller skating, was stunning.

Ryan also developed a close bond with his maternal grandparents, Tom and Gloria Hale. They often took care of Ryan and Andrea when Jeanne worked her shifts at Delco Electronics. In fact, Tom later credited his hospital-savvy grandson with saving his life. One morning, Tom had joined a relative for breakfast at a

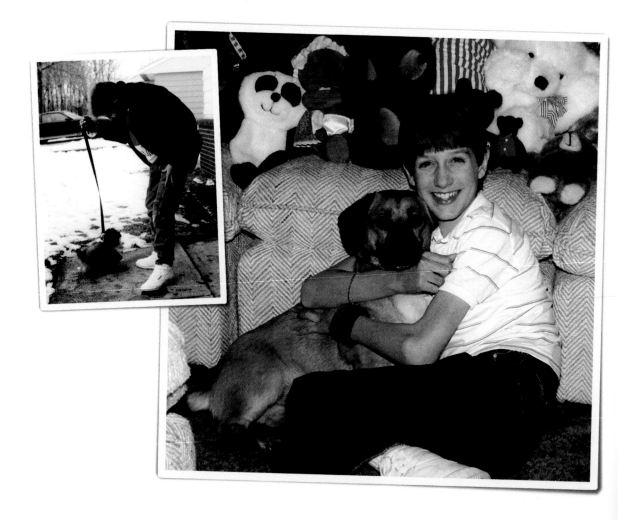

restaurant in Kokomo. On the way home, he began experiencing some alarming symptoms.

"When I got in the house, I told Gloria, 'My chest hurts, and I'm sweating something fierce,'" Tom recalled in an interview. "Sweat is pouring off me. Ryan was in the house with us. He spoke up and said, 'Grandpa, you're having a heart attack. You get to the hospital right now.'" Tom rushed to the hospital. It turned out Ryan was right. Doctors diagnosed a heart attack, and Tom quickly received proper treatment. "If he had not been there, I would have shrugged off those pains," Tom recalled several years after Ryan's death. "I might not be here today."

With his own health issues, Ryan could tell when he was about to experience what he and Jeanne called a "bleed," the pooling and eventual loss of blood, usually caused by unexpected physical contact with an object. His skin would tingle. Then, underlying vessels would swell. "As soon as he felt a bleed beginning, we could give him the Factor [VIII], and the bleed would stop," Jeanne recalled in her autobiography, *Weeding Out the Tears*. "But as he got older, he set his own agenda. If he thought the bleed and its treatment would keep him from doing something he really wanted to do, he wouldn't tell me about it. I'd get real mad when he did that."

With some of the more serious bleeding incidents, doctors ordered Ryan to wear Ace bandages. If his leg or knee were involved, he would be told to use crutches for three or four days. Just as he sometimes kept his bleeding symptoms from his mother, Ryan also did not always follow through with the bandages or crutches. "He didn't like kids saying, 'What's wrong with you now?'" Jeanne explained.

Although Ryan failed to disclose every aspect of his health and did not always follow doctor's orders, his fascination with medical issues was unwavering. For his tenth birthday, he asked his grandparents for a subscription to *Time* magazine. Ryan avidly read the health-related articles, then discussed them with his grandfather. The two began reading about AIDS, a frightening disorder spread by a virus. They learned that the virus is spread when an infected person has sexual relations with someone else because bodily fluids are exchanged. Experts also realized AIDS was being spread when drug users shared hypodermic needles contaminated with the virus.

Shortly before Ryan turned thirteen, his health took a turn for the worse. At night, he would wake up in a sweat. He began complaining about stomach pains. Sometimes he suddenly would get a fever, which would go away as mysteriously as it had come on. Increasingly worried, Jeanne took Ryan to a Kokomo clinic that served hemophiliacs. Health-care workers checked to make certain the Factor VIII was working properly.

Ryan's thirteenth birthday on December 6 passed uneventfully, but then came a crisis. "The next day, he got off the school bus, came in the house and said, 'Mom, you've got to do something,'" Jeanne recalled in *Weeding Out the Tears*. "I can't even get off the school bus without feeling tired.'" When his fever spiked at 104 degrees, Jeanne took him to the hospital. X-rays indicated he was suffering from pneumonia in both lungs. An ambulance rushed Ryan from Kokomo to Riley Hospital for Children in Indianapolis. At Riley, the Whites met Doctor Martin Kleiman, a highly regarded expert on infectious diseases in children.

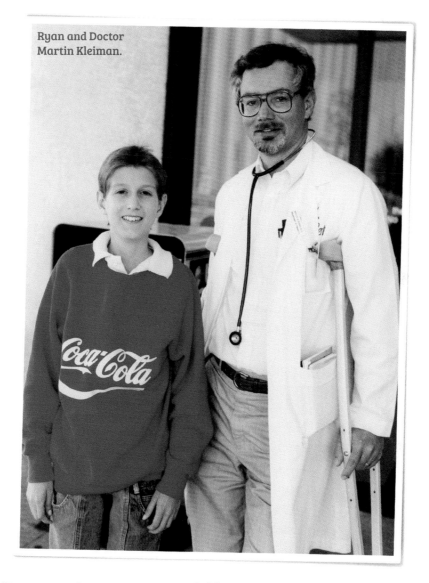

Ryan and Doctor Martin Kleiman.

"It was viral pneumonia, and I'd seen it in the cases of children with compromised immune systems for other reasons, such as tumors," Kleiman said. "I also knew it was an infection being seen with the HIV epidemic."

HIV is the virus that causes AIDS.

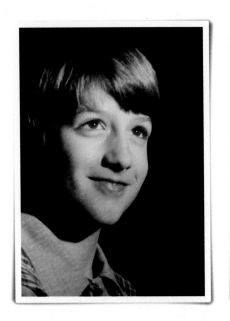
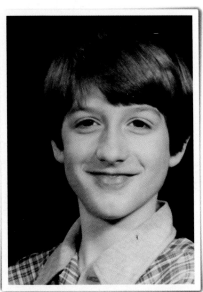
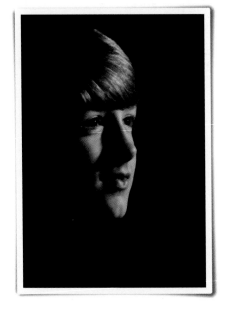
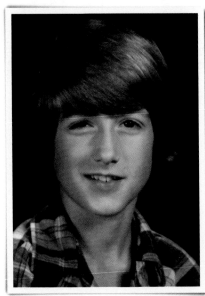

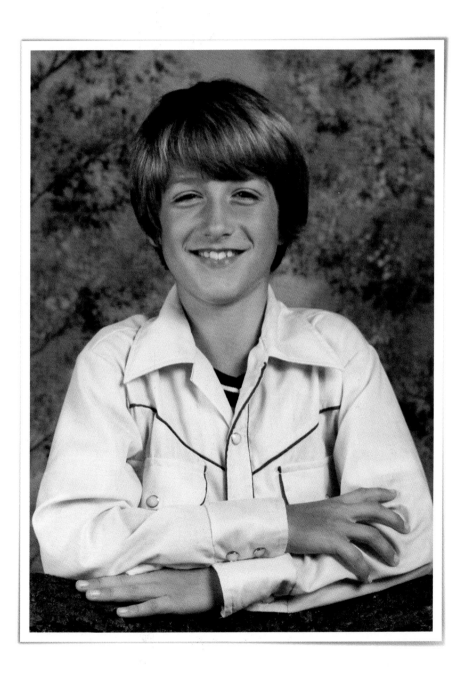

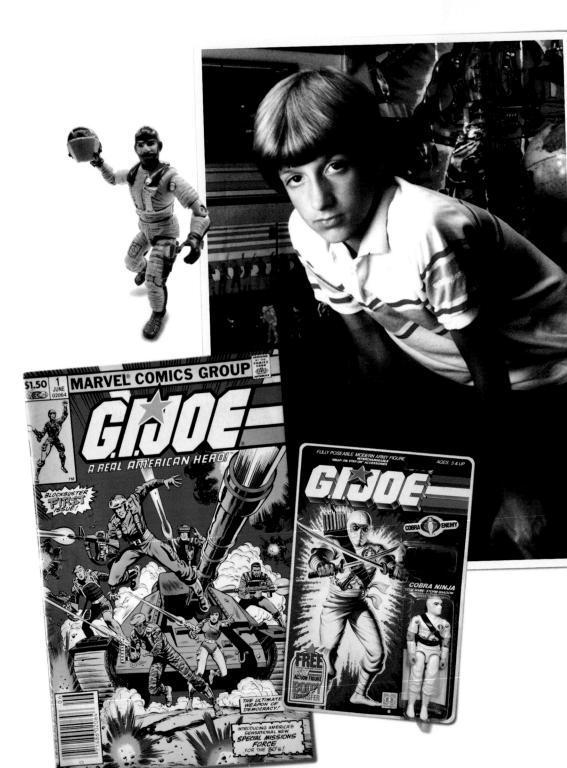

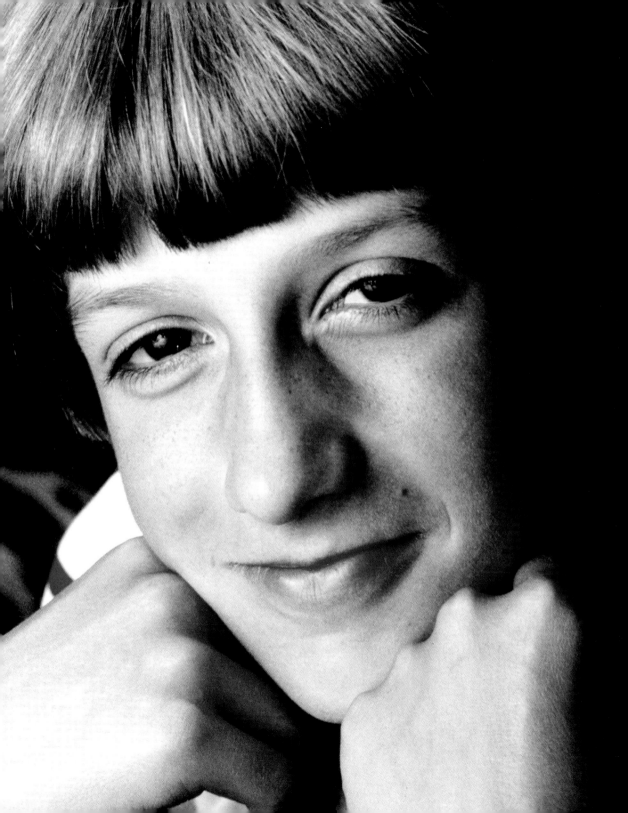

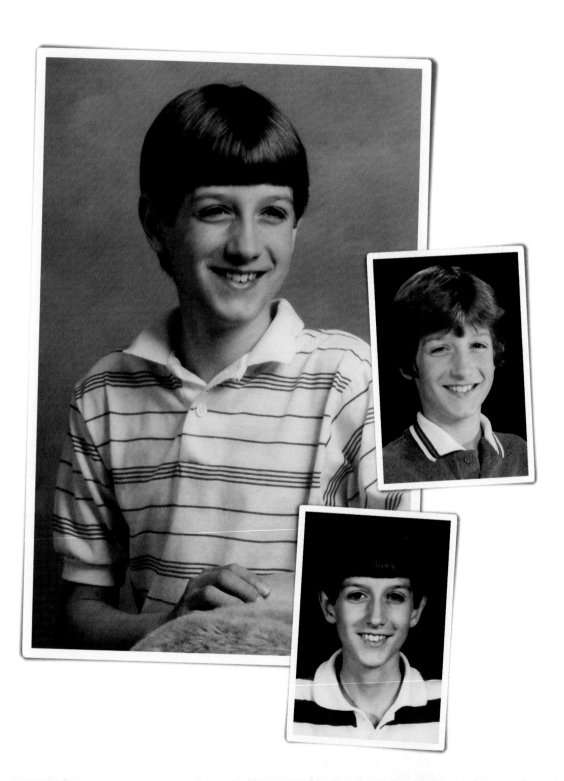

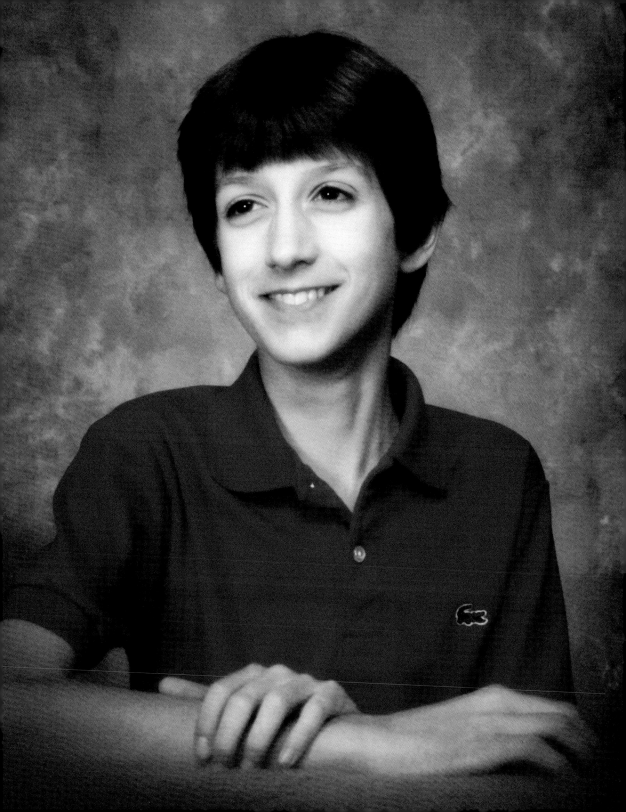

"I never wanted to be famous. It's embarrassing to be famous for being sick, especially with a disease like AIDS."

3

The diagnosis was devastating. At Riley Hospital for Children during the early days of the holiday season in 1984, Ryan was placed in isolation. Nurses, health-care workers, family, and friends were instructed to don gloves, masks, and gowns before visiting him. He was given about six months to live. "Six months was the generally recognized 'outside' estimate in 1984 with symptoms like Ryan presented," Doctor Martin Kleiman recalled in an interview years later.

Contaminated vials of Factor VIII, the blood-clotting agent for his hemophilia, were immediately identified as the source of the AIDS virus in Ryan. Recently he had been receiving even more injections of the factor than the two per week that had been routine. "Sometimes if he'd have a bleed, he'd get a shot every day for maybe thirty days," Jeanne recalled in her autobiography. "So he was probably infected not once, but thousands of times."

Rather than shuttle back and forth from Kokomo to Riley in Indianapolis, Jeanne and Andrea stayed across the street from the hospital in the Ronald McDonald House, a residence where relatives of Riley patients can live while their loved ones receive treatment.

On Christmas Day, as a result of treatment provided by Kleiman and other caregivers, Ryan began to improve. Tubes used to treat the pneumonia were removed. He was taken off a ventilator.

Jeanne was elated. But then, while she was eating breakfast at the Indiana University Medical Center, her mother, Gloria Hale, phoned with upsetting news.

The Whites' house in Kokomo had been burglarized. Gloria had dropped by to pick up some Christmas gifts and noticed a shattered window in the back door. Burglars had broken in and stolen all of the family's holiday presents as well as a videocassette recorder. Jeanne had purchased it for Andrea so she could study tapes of roller skating competitions. The burglars even had stolen videos of Andrea's dazzling routines during her earliest tournaments.

The burglary was completely unrelated to Ryan's AIDS diagnosis. (The news he was infected with the fatal disorder was known only to family members, health-care workers, and a few others.) Even so, the news was devastating. "My precious memories of my little girl's earliest skating meets, all gone," Jeanne recalled, referring to the stolen videos. "In the midst of this terrible crisis, my kids' Christmas had been stolen."

Jeanne went to Ryan's bedside at the hospital to break the news about the burglary to him. His new computer also had been stolen during the break-in. "All I said to Mom was, 'Let's forget about it.' I tried to think of the burglary as that book, *How the Grinch Stole Christmas*, come to life," he said in his autobiography.

When word of the Whites' misfortune spread through the hospital, they found themselves embraced by the holiday spirit.

Families of patients at Riley went to drugstores and bought Christmas gifts, including comic books and a remote-control model car for Ryan and a paint-by-numbers kit and popular Care Bears toys for Andrea. Their grandparents and other relatives arrived with cards and packages. Wayne dropped by with Izod shirts for Ryan. Even the hospital staff chipped in for gifts.

But there was devastating news far worse than the burglary to break to thirteen-year-old Ryan. Should he be told about the AIDS diagnosis and his life expectancy? Jeanne was hesitant, but several other family members, including Wayne, emphasized Ryan needed to know. News that Ryan was infected with the frightening, fatal disorder was bound to get out and spread, they argued. He should learn about the diagnosis from his loved ones, not from gossip.

So on the day after Christmas, Jeanne and Andrea came to Ryan's hospital room accompanied by a minister. Jeanne explained that the series of tests at Riley had determined he had AIDS. Ryan's reaction showed no signs of panic. But he immediately offered up a game plan: "Let's just pretend that I don't have it." Just as instantly, Jeanne explained that would not be possible. It was unrealistic. Precautions needed to be taken for Ryan.

Fortunately, Ryan's recovery from pneumonia continued. Even in the hospital in early January, he began talking about returning to school. Kleiman said he had no reservations about risks to classmates and teachers. "Even then, it was abundantly clear that there needed to be an exchange of bodily fluids for infection to occur," he recalled.

To a frightened public, medical experts emphasized that AIDS could not be transmitted by sharing a water fountain, drinking

"Mom had taught me to look
for the happy parts of life, and to
look away from the bad parts."

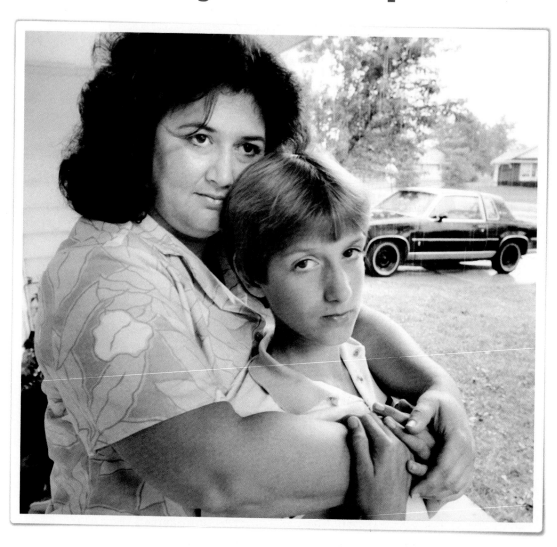

from the same glass, or any sort of casual contact. AIDS, they repeatedly stressed, was transmitted through sexual contact, sharing infected needles, or receiving contaminated blood products such as the Factor VIII used to treat Ryan's hemophilia. Not only did Ryan pose no danger to classmates and teachers, Kleiman said, but he also never worried about the reverse situation, that someone at school could infect Ryan with an illness that would dangerously weaken him. "There was no risk to Ryan that wasn't worth taking—the risks were so incredibly small," said Kleiman.

Ryan explained it this way in *My Own Story*: "Hemophilia had taught me I was always going to have to go for it—to concentrate on all the things I wanted to do. Mom had taught me to look for the happy parts of life, and to look away from the bad parts. If I had started dwelling on all the bad stuff connected with the hemophilia, I'd never have left the hospital at all. I didn't want to *have* AIDS, I wanted to *fight* it. I wasn't going to be an AIDS *victim*. No one was going to make any kind of victim out of me."

On January 24, 1985, Ryan was discharged from Riley Hospital. He returned with his family to their Kokomo home on South Webster Street. Although Ryan was feeble and weighed less than sixty pounds, he was regaining strength.

Other good news awaited Jeanne, who had been feeling overwhelmed by bills related to the treatment of a catastrophic illness. After the robbery, her coworkers at Delco Electronics had taken up a collection to help pay bills not covered by insurance, including her mortgage, car payment, gasoline, and food.

Regarding food, Kleiman's instructions to Jeanne were to do anything possible to persuade Ryan to eat. He always had been finicky, but he loved certain things, including Denny's beef stew, hot chocolate from Wendy's restaurants, pizza, and his grandmother's meat loaf. Jeanne and Gloria spent a lot of time in the kitchen,

While Ryan was recovering at home, news about his AIDS diagnosis spread throughout Kokomo and Russiaville. The sources of the whispers were unclear, but acquaintances and even strangers obviously were learning about the diagnosis of the terrifying, misunderstood disorder. For the Whites, the first, ominous clues came when they noticed that restaurant managers in the Kokomo area were tossing their dishes and silverware in garbage cans and dumpsters after they left.

Initially, Jeanne was not too bothered by the overreactions. She was delighted to notice Ryan's more robust health, which included a weight gain. She also received support when she contacted organizations such as the American Foundation for AIDS Research and shared the news about Ryan. "Andrea helped by making Mom and me posters with fancy lettering that said, 'Number One Brother' or 'Love You Mom,'" Ryan recalled in his autobiography. "She also got chores done after Mom asked her to do them only once—something you can almost never say about her."

Andrea also continued competing in skating tournaments. Family friends took her to practices and competitions so Jeanne could stay home with Ryan. Jeanne also frequently brought him to a Kokomo hospital for various treatments, as well as to Riley Hospital for visits with Kleiman.

As the winter of 1985 continued, news about Ryan snowballed. Media outlets, including the *CBS Morning News*, began phoning Jeanne. She did not deny that her son had AIDS. Later, she wrote that she was too naïve to consider trying to cover up the health issues. Strangers, including scores of preachers, immediately began phoning the Whites with suggestions about "cures." Others mailed letters. In one, the letter writer urged Ryan to eat five walnuts daily for twenty-one consecutive days. Other letters urged Ryan to fast.

Ryan analyzed the reaction this way: "Often, the next letter I read contradicted the previous one." The suggestion that he fast, he said, was conveying the absurd notion that, as he put it, "I was supposed to starve myself to get well."

Amid all of this, Ryan started, as Jeanne put it, "bugging" her about returning to Western Middle School and attending classes with his friends. Uncertain about what to do, Jeanne tried to avoid the issue. Ryan, though, persisted with his pleas. So, at the end of March 1985, the day before the school's spring break, Jeanne contacted Ron Colby, Western Middle School principal. She indicated that Ryan would like to return to school on a day when the students would be enjoying a pizza lunch.

Colby's relationship with the Whites had been amicable. Long before the AIDS diagnosis, there had been consultations between him and the school nurse about how to handle issues related to Ryan's severe hemophilia, the bleeding disorder. "What if he falls in PE class? What if he gets bumped in the hallway?" Colby said in an interview years later, recalling the questions that needed to be addressed. "We informed teachers that Ryan could bleed internally and that symptoms might include a large bruise."

Now, with the diagnosis of AIDS, there were new, even more complicated issues to consider and work through. With spring break imminent, Colby suggested that Jeanne wait and contact him after classes resumed.

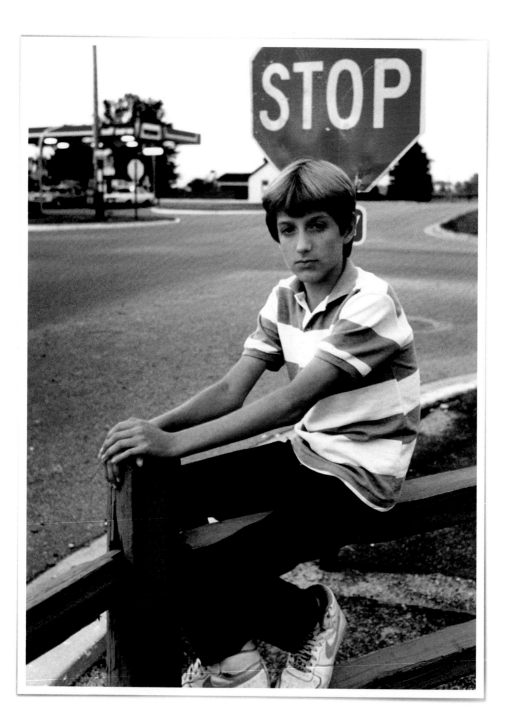

Agreeing, Jeanne decided the family should take a vacation to Alabama to visit her sister, Janet, and her family. The warm weather seemed to help Ryan gain even more vigor. During that trip, Ryan played with his cousins, rode a bicycle, and enjoyed plenty of other activities.

After the family's return to Kokomo, Ryan continued to mention how much he wanted to return to school. Still unsure how to proceed, Jeanne got in touch again with Colby and inquired about various options, including ways Ryan could receive home-based instruction. Then, because the school year was winding down, she told Colby it probably was too late to launch any new program. Jeanne indicated she would be back in touch with him during the summer.

By then, the principal had been informed by Howard County health officials that Ryan should not be readmitted to Western Middle School.

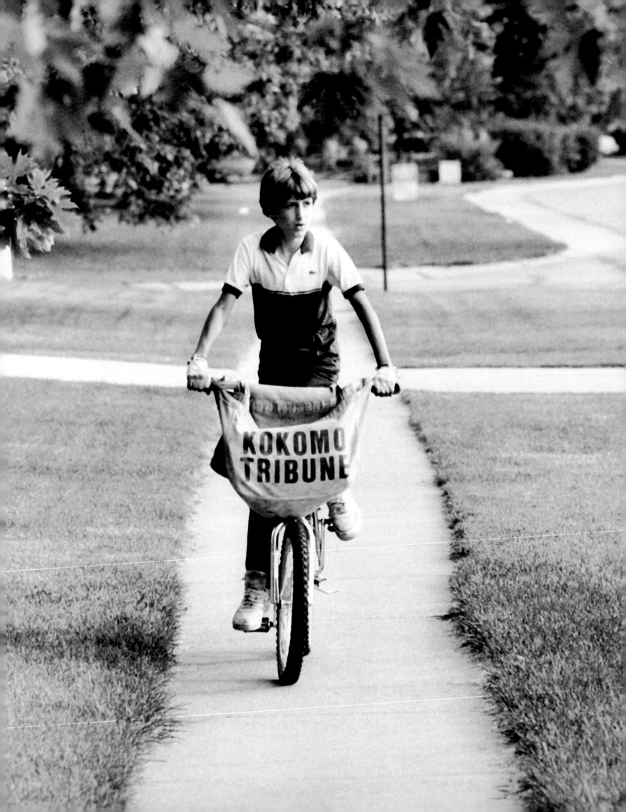

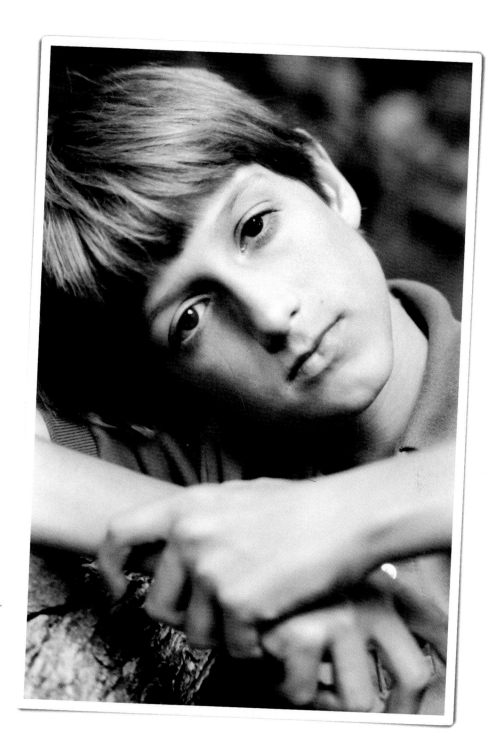

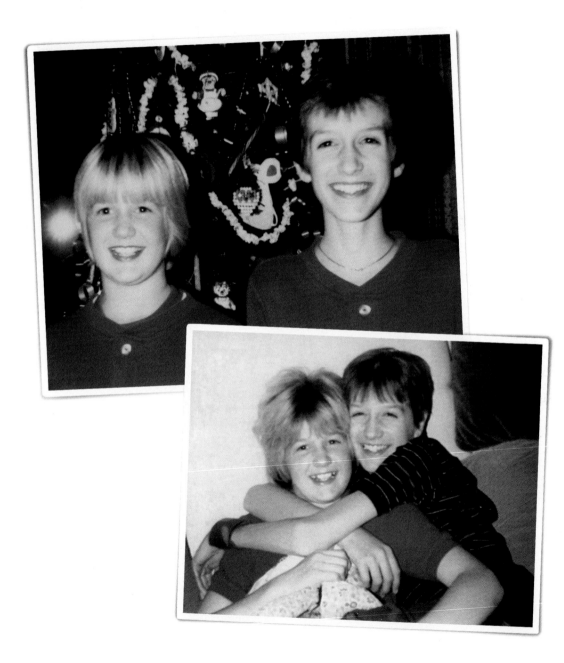

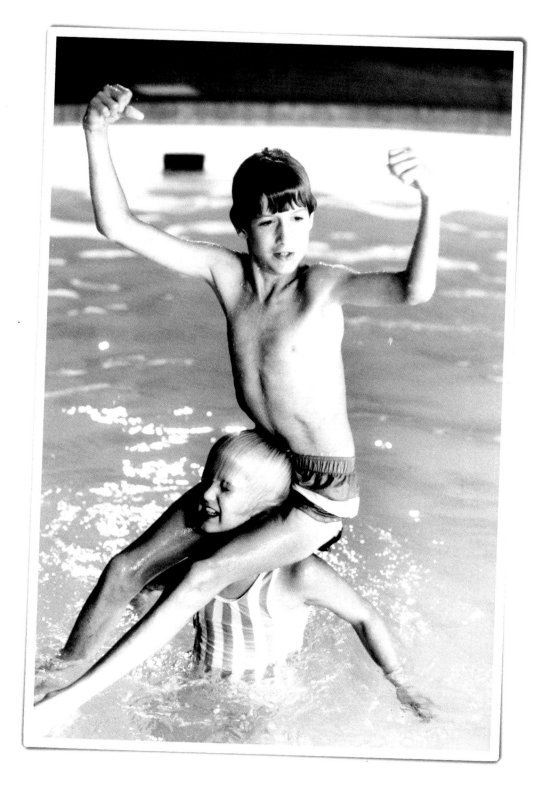

"Sometimes I was scared and upset, and it came out in tears. . . . Other times I didn't cry; I got mad."

4

In 1985 state regulations left decision making up to health officials in each of Indiana's ninety-two counties about whether or not local schools should admit students with potentially contagious diseases. Parents who objected to decisions by the local county officials had no way to appeal them. (As a result of Ryan White's crusade, Indiana Health Commissioner Woodrow Myers instructed his staff to lobby state legislators to change the regulations so that an appeal process would be available. That change eventually occurred, one of several ramifications of Ryan's case.)

In late July, administrators at Western School Corporation announced that Ryan would not be readmitted to school in the fall. Risks to other students were too uncertain, they explained. School officials also said they had been frustrated when requesting practical, detailed guidelines from the Indiana Department of Health about how to deal with a wide range of situations that could occur with an AIDS-infected student in hallways, classrooms, cafeterias, and restrooms.

Howard County school administrators said state health officials moved too slowly to get guidelines to them. Even when initial guidelines were received, the administrators charged, the guidelines were too broad or vague to be helpful in dealing with specific challenges that could arise during a hectic school day, such as what

kind of disinfectant to use if a student with AIDS fell, endured
a cut, or bled for any other reason. When guidelines finally were
received, there was not enough time for Western Middle School
to react and implement precautionary procedures, Dan Carter,
president of the school board, said during an interview.

Ryan was shattered to learn he would be prohibited from
attending school with his friends. He informed his mother they
should challenge the decision. In his autobiography, Ryan wrote
that he told Jeanne, "We *have* to fight, Mom. If we don't, we won't
be allowed to go anywhere or do anything. What they want to do
isn't right."

By then, national media, including morning television news
programs, were picking up on the controversy in Indiana. Programs
such as *Good Morning, America* on ABC contacted the Whites and
asked them to make appearances.

At his office in downtown Indianapolis, Myers decided he
needed to intervene and take a forceful, public stand. A tall, husky
man with a commanding presence, he had grown up in the Hoosier
capital and graduated from Shortridge High School when he was
just sixteen years old. After graduating from Stanford University
when he was only nineteen, he received his medical training from
the renowned Harvard Medical School.

When the controversy about Ryan began unfolding in 1985,
Myers had only been back in Indiana for a few months. He had
been on the medical staff at a hospital in San Francisco, where
many of the earliest cases of AIDS were reported. At San Francisco
General Hospital, where Myers worked in the intensive care unit,
"We probably had more patients with AIDS than any other hospital

in the country," he recalled. "I certainly had more experience in
dealing with AIDS than any other physician in Indiana in 1985."

In early 1985 Indiana governor Robert Orr appointed Myers
as the state health commissioner, even though the governor was a
Republican and Myers was a Democrat. So Myers, who was known
as Woody to his Indiana friends and acquaintances, returned to his
home state.

Galvanized by the news about Western School Corporation's
refusal to admit a fourteen-year-old boy with AIDS, Myers
sent guidelines to the school, emphasizing that Ryan should be
readmitted and that no danger existed to him or others as long
as certain precautions were taken. He also made inquiries about
the White family's schedule. Learning in early August they would
be returning from an appearance on a morning televsion show
based in New York City, he decided to
meet Jeanne and Ryan, and introduce
himself, when they disembarked at
Indianapolis International Airport.

"I decided we should use the bully
pulpit to put pressure on Howard
County," he recalled. After introducing
himself to the Whites, Myers
explained that he wanted to hold a
press conference with them at his side,
emphasizing that Ryan should be in
school. The Whites agreed.

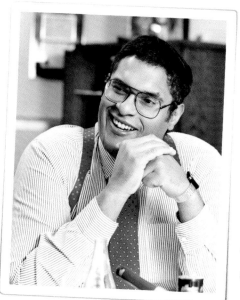

INDIANAPOLIS STAR

Doctor Woodrow Myers.

Recalling the press conference years later, Myers said he wanted to add a touch of humanity. He also wanted to visually demonstrate the lack of any reason to fear contact with Ryan, and to reinforce the boy's young age and engaging personality. "So I deliberately tousled his hair as I spoke," he said. "Ryan was extremely poised for a kid his age. He just stuck to his line. 'I want to go to school like a normal kid.'"

In the Kokomo area, many felt Myers had inflamed the situation by interjecting himself. "Woody Myers went high-profile, using the most pejorative terms," said Carter. "It was clear to us that he was seeking the stage and the spotlight."

By mid-August, parents of more than a hundred Howard County children signed forms threatening a civil suit if Ryan was allowed back in school. Several dozen teachers in the area indicated they supported the decision to keep Ryan out. Charles Vaughan Sr., a Lafayette-based attorney who had represented adult AIDS patients with various legal issues, contacted the Whites. A forceful, persuasive lawyer not known for backing down from a challenge, Vaughan assured Jeanne and Ryan that they could achieve the legal right for him to return to school. "He also said, 'Ryan, this could get ugly,'" Jeanne recalled. "Ryan just said, "I can take it.'"

At Western, teachers met ten days before the start of fall classes. Fifty of them voted to support the administration's decision to bar Ryan from returning to school. Two voted in favor of allowing him to come back. Petitions circulated among the students and parents. Although dozens of signatures were collected on a petition that advocated barring Ryan from school, a counterpetition drive, led by Western student Wanda Bowen, was signed by more than two hundred people in the community, sympathizing with the Whites and supporting Ryan's return.

As classes began at Western without Ryan, administrators consulted with the Whites and various teachers about ways he could learn the seventh-grade curriculum even if he was not in the classroom. An interactive, audio-only device was hooked up that worked through the phone lines, connecting teachers and students with Ryan at home. The technical device included a microphone in the classroom and resembled a yardstick. (This was many years before Skype and other, sophisticated interactive devices were available. Even e-mail was not yet widely available.)

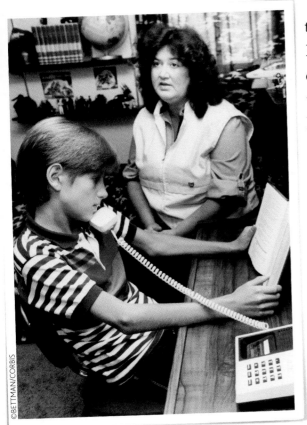

Ryan never liked the telephone hookup situation. In his autobiography, he complained that the audio was weak. He often could not hear his classmates. Sometimes even the teachers' voices faded, particularly when they moved around the classroom as they spoke. Ron Colby, the school's principal, conceded there were some initial challenges with the interactive device. But they were quickly resolved within a day or two, he noted.

©BETTMAN/CORBIS

Teachers and administrators, he emphasized, remained sensitive to Ryan's instructional needs. As an example, Colby recalled a day when teachers notified him they were not receiving responses from Ryan. "I got in my car and drove to the Whites' house," he said. "It turned out Ryan was playing with his Army people (GI Joes). What do you expect? He was a kid. It was no big deal, but I mention it to indicate the attention and effort involved on our part."

Jeanne, though, said the technical problems with the interactive device persisted longer than just a few days. Several different types of hookups between the classroom and the Whites' home were installed through the phone lines, she said.

As autumn continued, Ryan kept lobbying to return to the classroom with his friends and peers. At get togethers after school, though, some friends told him they could not continue to see him. Their parents had objections or concerns, they explained. Other friends stuck by Ryan despite intense peer pressure. One of Ryan's best friends was called ugly names, including "fag," for maintaining his friendship with Ryan. "It hurts—I won't pretend it doesn't," Jeanne acknowledged.

The Whites, their friends, health officials, and reporters also began hearing rumors that Ryan had been seen spitting on vegetables in supermarkets or trying to spread the AIDS virus in other ways. None of the rumors were verified or determined to have a shred of truth.

Ryan's health took some turns for the worse in the fall of 1985. Periodically running fevers and coughing, he was admitted to Riley Children's Hospital. Once again, there were some positive results from the hospitalization, at least from Ryan's perspective. He began receiving letters of support and gifts from across the country and even beyond. Some came from as far away as Russia.

In late November, a hearing officer for the Indiana Department of Education ruled that Ryan must be admitted to school. A few weeks later, the Western District School Board unanimously voted to appeal the ruling. "We still didn't have a certificate from the county health official saying he was able to attend school," Carter recalled years later. "That was required under the law at the time. We felt we had to uphold the law."

Reacting to the controversy, a group called Concerned Citizens of Kokomo formed. The group supported the decision to keep Ryan out of Western Middle School.

The controversy also divided neighbors and churches, including the congregation at a Methodist church the Whites attended. According to Ryan, many congregation members even refused to shake his hand during moments of fellowship. Others in the community expressed support; they included the *Kokomo Tribune*, which published an editorial supporting Ryan's crusade to attend school.

At the state board of health, Myers and his staff started planning outreach, educational programs about AIDS. Nurse practitioners and other staff members prepared to visit communities and schools across the state. "We wanted to explain how AIDS was transmitted—and how it was *not*," said Lou Ann Baker, AIDS education coordinator for the Board of Health. "We met with Jeanne and Ryan. She was in a reactive mode, as most mothers would be, and she usually did most of the talking. Ryan would kick her ankle if he didn't agree with what she was saying."

Doctor Martin Kleiman said, "It was unequivocably clear even then that you could not acquire HIV without the transfer of bodily fluids. Overwhelming amounts of information was coming to the public from reliable sources. The challenge was that it's hard to teach people who are so fearful."

A delegation representing the State Board of Health met with Carter and other Western school officials to recommend Ryan be readmitted. "I said to them, 'Gentleman, you have heard the law on communicable diseases and the requirement that the county health official certify a student,'" Carter recalled. "I said, 'In light of this law, how do you reconcile your recommendation that we go ahead and admit him to school?' They said, 'We can't.'"

The stalemate continued until February 1986, when an appeals board at the Indiana Department of Education ruled Ryan should be allowed to attend school. Health officials in Howard County then certified that he was fit to return to the classroom. Colby said extensive preparations were made for his return. Educators felt confident they could handle any problems that arose.

Ryan showed up on Friday, February 21, for one day of class. Of the 360 sixth and seventh graders at Western, 151 were absent, or 43 percent. Despite the much higher than normal absenteeism, the first day of Ryan's return went well. Colby told reporters that Ryan's fellow students "accepted" him. "They talked with him. They patted him on the back and welcomed him back."

Although there were no restrictions about where Ryan could sit in class, he used a separate restroom (the faculty restroom) and ate with disposable lunch utensils. When Ryan left the school after his final class, he told reporters that his return was "a lot of fun. I'm glad to be back."

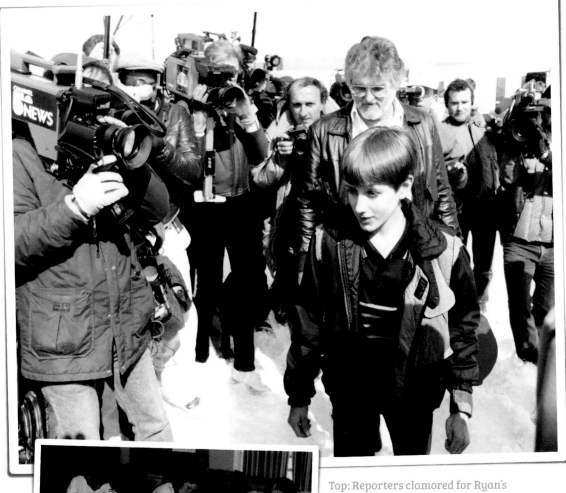

Top: Reporters clamored for Ryan's attention during his return to school. Left: Ryan at his desk in English class at Western Middle School.

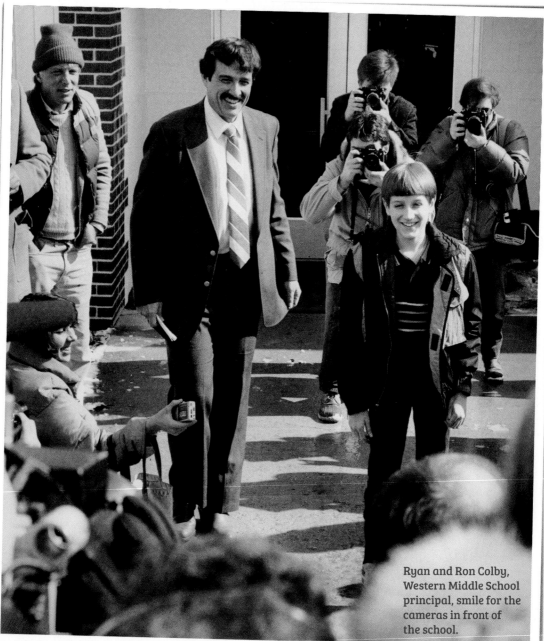

Ryan and Ron Colby, Western Middle School principal, smile for the cameras in front of the school.

However, that Friday turned out to be his only day in class for a while. Later that day, the Concerned Citizens group secured a restraining order from a Howard County Circuit Court that, at least temporarily, would keep Ryan out of school. "That was probably the worst day of my life," Colby said years later. "We had made such extensive preparations, so it was devastating to have all of this unresolved."

The principal expressed no regrets on another front, though. Myers, Baker, and others contended that, unlike other Indiana communities, Western school officials turned down their offers to host AIDS education forums in the community. "By that point, the community had so much disdain for the State Board of Health officials that it would have been counterproductive," Colby said.

In early April, the restraining order from the Howard County Circuit Court was dissolved by a higher court. Ryan was able to return to school on April 10. On that day, twenty-seven students at Western stayed home. Then, a group of parents announced the opening of a private school in Russiaville for families who did not want their children to attend classes with Ryan.

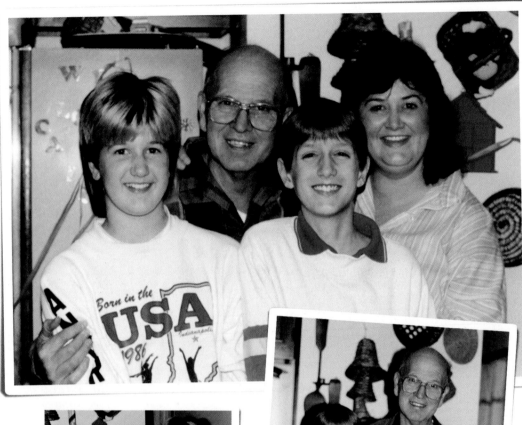
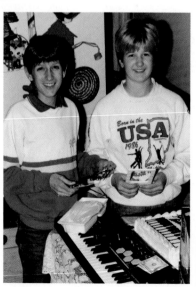
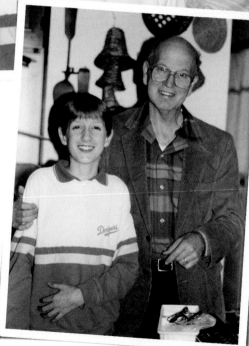

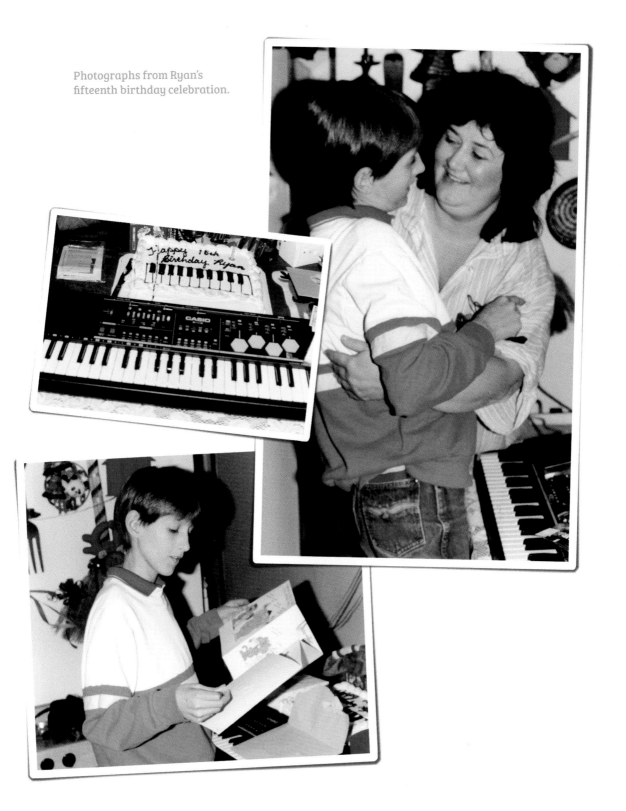

Photographs from Ryan's fifteenth birthday celebration.

"Sometimes I make people nervous because I look so young. I stopped growing when I was twelve, thanks to AIDS."

5

The White family found beer cans, fast-food cartons, whiskey bottles, and other trash on the lawn of their house on Webster Street in Kokomo. Not just once or twice, but frequently enough that cleaning up garbage in the grass became routine. With trash bags in hand, Jeanne, Ryan, and Andrea White took turns picking up the mess.

Almost unbelievably, though, trash dumps were offset by offers of support from celebrities Ryan and Jeanne never dreamed of meeting. Among the most outspoken was international rock star Elton John, who had been enjoying spectacular successes as a singer-composer for nearly fifteen years.

A remark by Ryan during an appearance on the ABC-TV news program *Good Morning, America* inadvertently led to the family's friendship with the British-born entertainer. He already was famous for such songs as "Goodbye Yellow Brick Road," "Don't Go Breaking My Heart," "Rocket Man," "Daniel," "Crocodile Rock," and countless other hits. Ryan appeared on the morning news show after he was asked to attend a glittering event in New York City to raise money for AIDS research. Celebrities such as Academy Award–winning movie star Elizabeth Taylor, fashion designer Calvin Klein, and television actress Marlo Thomas also planned to attend. On *Good Morning, America*, Ryan was asked which celebrity he most looked forward to meeting at the gala. "Elton John," he replied. "Definitely Elton John."

Jeanne recalled, "Ryan always said he liked Elton John because he was comfortable with being different from everyone else." John was known for his flashy outfits and oversized sunglasses.

Much to Ryan's disappointment, though, he did not meet the rock star at the fund-raiser for the American Foundation for AIDS Research. During the gala and at preevent publicity appearances for it, Ryan spent hours posing for photos with countless other celebrities. Responding to requests, he even posed with the cast of the Broadway musical *Cats*. But his music idol did not show up. As it turned out, John was unable to attend because he was recovering from jet lag.

The next morning, AmFar arranged for a limo to pick up Ryan, Jeanne, and Andrea at their New York hotel and whisk them to the airport. En route, a phone for the limo service rang in the car. The caller was John, who apologized for missing the celebrity fund-raiser, but reported he had seen Ryan talk about him on television. The rock singer promised to keep in contact with the Whites and to bring them as his guests to upcoming concerts.

Other celebrities also began contacting the Whites, including country singer Ronnie Milsap and televison actor David Hasselhoff, who sent T-shirts. So did the Harvard Medical School. Olympic diver Greg Louganis, who already was being regarded as the best diver in competitive history after winning both of the gold medals available in his sport at the 1984 Los Angeles Summer Olympic Games, contacted the Whites to express support. Televison talk show host Phil Donahue also extended help, publicly and privately.

In response, some accused the Whites of reveling in the attention and complained that Jeanne was a stage mother, manipulating the crisis for fame. Many close to the family, though, emphasized the reverse was the case. They said Jeanne merely was following her son's wishes, subverting her desire to end the controversy and its disruption of her family's life because Ryan desperately wanted to be in school.

He may have been only four feet, eleven inches tall and weighed seventy-six pounds in the spring of 1986—definitely on the short,

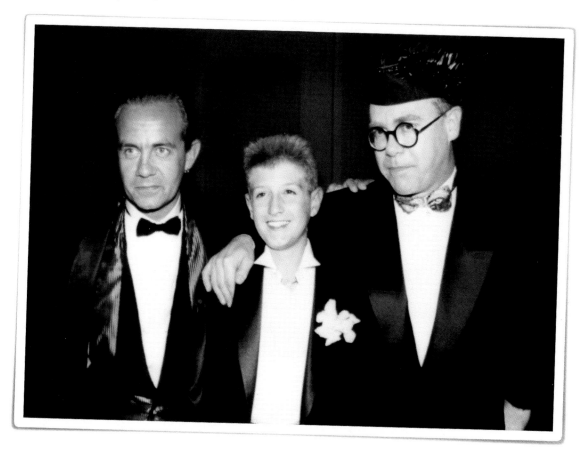

Ryan poses with (left) Bernie Taupin and Elton John at a children's benefit in Los Angeles.

scrawny side for a fourteen-year-old boy—but he always made his presence felt in family decisions, according to people who interacted with the Whites. "Ryan White is the man in that house," Charles Vaughan Sr., the Lafayette lawyer who helped the family in the battle to get Ryan reinstated in school, said in an interview. "A decision that affects Ryan is made by Ryan. He absolutely calls all the shots. Every time you ask Jeanne anything, she looks at Ryan for the decision as to what to do." At Western Middle School, Ron Colby agreed. "I personally do not have the opinion that Jeanne is a stage mother. She is a working parent in a single-parent household. She does what she thinks her son wants."

Meanwhile, during the spring of 1986 about two dozen students were attending class at the Russiaville Home Study School, the private school formed by families who did not want their children interacting with Ryan. The school conducted classes in a former American Legion hall.

At Western, Ryan often felt isolated, he wrote in his autobiography. "Other kids backed up against their lockers when they saw me coming, or they threw themselves against the hallway walls, shouting, 'Watch out! Watch out! There he is!'"

Ryan seldom talked back, even when he had increasing opportunities with the escalating media attention. Jeanne frequently asked her son how he kept from getting upset about the hostile reactions of some people in the community. "He'd say, 'Mom, they're just trying to protect their own kids the way you're trying to protect me.'"

During an interview at the Whites' house, a feature writer for the *Indianapolis News* asked Jeanne why the family did not simply

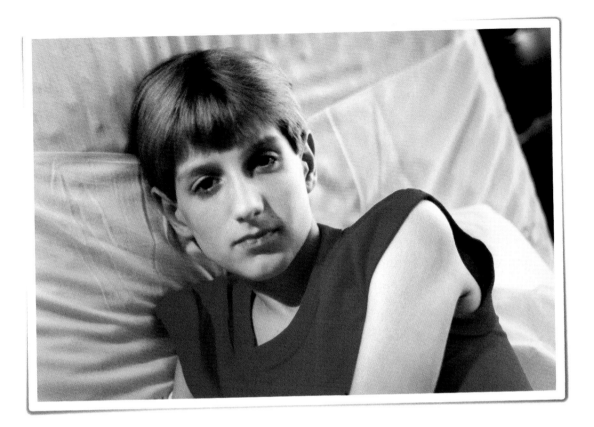

move from Kokomo. In response, Jeanne looked the journalist directly in the eye. "So who," she asked, "will buy 'the AIDS house'?"

The break for summer brought its own challenges. If Ryan spent a day in the sun, large red blotches would appear on his skin. The blotches, which showed up across his body, did not just alarm Jeanne. They also scared Ryan, who usually tried not to admit to fears. On some nights, he endured high fevers and sweats. Sometimes he also was bothered by a hacking cough.

After school resumed in August, Ryan was in and out of the hospital to treat his various health challenges. His hospital stays meant Jeanne and other family members frequently could not take Andrea to roller skating practices. She missed so many practices— often because, with few complaints, she accompanied Jeanne and Ryan to the hospital—that Andrea eventually announced she intended to give up competitive roller skating. Her lack of practice meant she was being surpassed by girls whom she used to beat regularly. Although Jeanne expressed disappointment that her daughter's roller skating career had to end because of Ryan's health issues, she acknowledged Andrea's decision was the sensible approach.

John provided a big boost by sending airplane tickets to Southern California for Ryan, Jeanne, and Andrea. The trip included a personal tour of Disneyland, courtesy of the rock star. During the tour, Ryan occasionally was too weak to walk. The group fetched a wheelchair, and the international rock star volunteered to push. Continually displaying what Jeanne later described as unflagging "energy and good nature," John wheeled Ryan around at speeds that delighted the young Hoosier. Under the California sun, Ryan even developed a slight tan—not red splotches.

"I wanted to give him an adventure—limos, planes, fancy hotels—a carefree time to take his mind off his difficult circumstances," John recalled in his memoir about the impact of the AIDS epidemic on his life. "But what I remember most about that visit is that I had at least as much fun as Ryan, if not more." At that point, the pop superstar later revealed, he was addicted to cocaine and frequently indulged his temper, throwing fits over trivialities such as the color of the curtains in his hotel rooms. "Ryan, on the other hand, was dying," John noted. "His family had been tormented. And yet, during his trip to L.A. and every time I

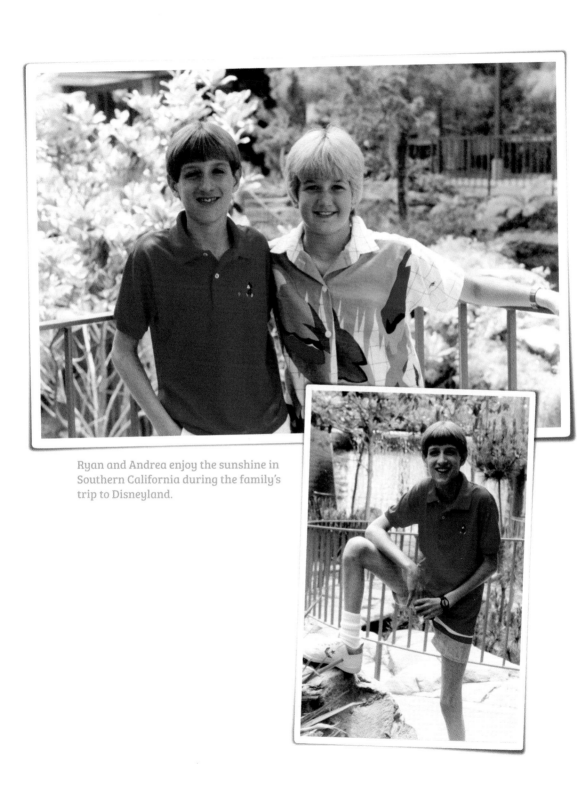

Ryan and Andrea enjoy the sunshine in Southern California during the family's trip to Disneyland.

was with him from then on, he was so relentlessly upbeat."

The excitement for the Whites continued after they returned home from Disneyland. Louganis notified them he would be competing in the national championships of USA Diving, which is headquartered in Indianapolis. Louganis invited the family to be his guests during the competition at the Indiana University Natatorium, which had been the site of the 1984 U.S. Olympic Trials.

Not only did Louganis begin telling reporters that he considered Ryan a "hero," when the muscular athlete won the national championship, as expected, he also gave the medal to Ryan. Louganis even urged Ryan to climb the steps to the top of the 10-meter platform, commonly known as the "high dive." Although Ryan did not jump off, just the climb—and the panoramic view from high above the spectacular pool—was thrilling.

Such highs were followed by frequent lows. Ryan complained he discovered vicious, antihomosexual slurs written on his folders and binders in his locker at school. Instead of throwing out the folders, Jeanne kept them as evidence of the torment that confronted her son.

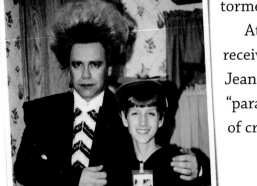

At home the Whites continued to receive a steady stack of hate mail. Jeanne conceded she began to feel "paranoid" because of the bombardment of criticisms and rumors about her son

Ryan meets with Elton John at the singer's 1986 concert in Oakland, California.

spitting on supermarket vegetables and fruit. She even learned about gossip that Ryan had deliberately cut himself to spread the disease. The notion that Ryan, whose lifelong hemophilia had posed such challenges for him, would deliberately slice at himself was outrageous to the family. Recalling the volatile situation years later, Doctor Martin Kleiman said, "There are a lot of people in the Kokomo area who should say, 'I was wrong. I am so sorry for the way we reacted.'"

Although Ryan never wavered in his determination to keep going to school, he admitted he was, as he put it, "desperate" to live in a different community. The Whites, though, felt trapped because of the inability to sell their Kokomo house and buy a new house elsewhere. Then, there were a couple of surprises.

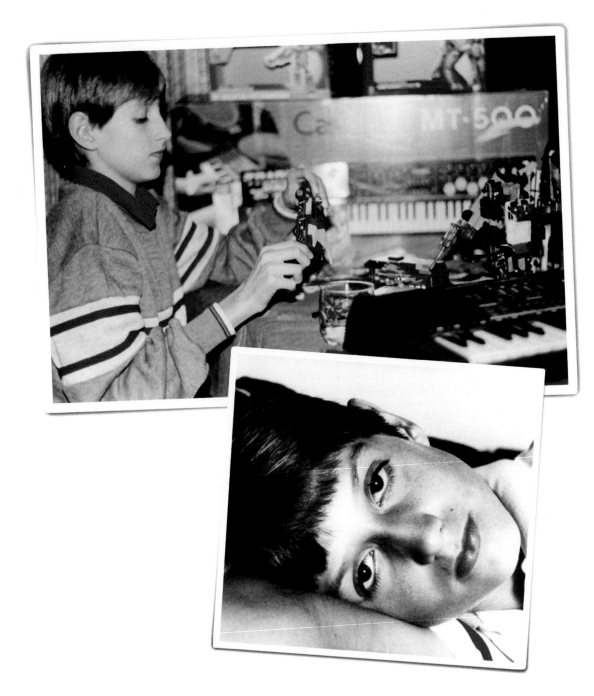

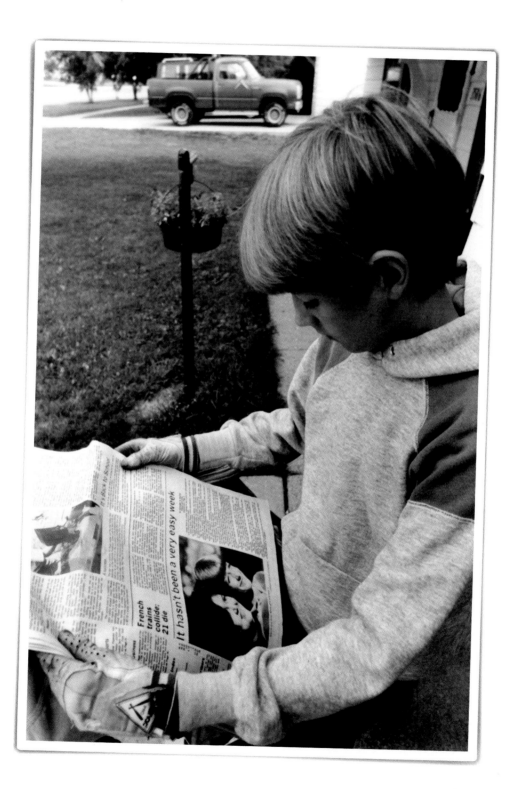

When a kid asked him if he would give up his fame to get rid of AIDS, Ryan responded: "How dumb can you get! I snapped my fingers at him. 'Like that," I said. 'I'd give it up like that.'"

6

A production company based in Southern California contacted the Whites. The producers wanted to make a television-movie about Ryan's life. For the TV movie, which was to be called the *Ryan White Story*, the family would be paid for the use of his name and for advice in the script and filming.

That infusion of funds, along with an offer of a cash gift from Elton John, meant Jeanne could afford to make a down payment on a new house in a different community. In John's memoir about the impact of the AIDS epidemic on his life, the pop superstar revealed he intended to send money to Jeanne as a gift. "But Jeanne absolutely insisted on a loan. In fact, she made both of us sign a homemade contract stating that she would pay me back. Sure enough, years later I received a check from Jeanne," recalled John.

The Whites embarked on house hunting. Eventually the family decided to move about twenty-five miles south of Kokomo to the lakeside town of Cicero in Hamilton County. The Whites moved into their new home, a two-story, Cape Cod-style house, in May 1987. The new house was located on Lake Cicero. A small woods was nearby. Although Ryan and Andrea were ecstatic, Jeanne worried about the community reaction. "I didn't want to seem to be sneaking into Hamilton County," she recalled in her book *Weeding Out the Tears*.

She contacted the county's health officials as well as Hamilton Heights High School, which Ryan would be attending in the fall, to alert them about the family's move. Many of her fears were quickly dispelled. Almost as soon as the Whites settled in their new home, neighbors rang their doorbell to welcome them.

Among the first Cicero neighbors to greet them was the family of Betsy and Jim Stewart, who lived two doors away. The Stewarts' seventeen-year-old daughter, Jill Stewart, an incoming senior at Hamilton Heights, had been elected student body president. Along with many of her classmates, she had followed reports about Ryan's crusade to attend school in Kokomo. "It was national news, and most of us were saying, 'Wow, it's understandable for a community to be afraid, but the whole thing wasn't handled as well as it could be,'" Jill recalled in an interview years later. "We felt a lot of empathy for Ryan. Then, he moved to our community—two doors down from my family. We went over to their house with food to welcome them. I bonded immediately with Ryan and Jeanne."

Doctor Woodrow Myers, the state health commissioner, realized the family's move to a new community offered a fresh opportunity. By attending a different school, Ryan would be in the spotlight again and this time, with proper planning, his attendance could be far less polarizing. "I realized we had a moment to create a success story," Myers recalled.

Jill and other teenagers at Hamilton Heights could become role models in responding to people with AIDS in their midst, Myers and other health and civic officials decided. After conferring with Doctor Otis Bown, a former Indiana governor and physician who was serving as U.S. Secretary of Health and Human Services, Myers concluded that Ryan's classmates and other Hamilton Heights students could calm their parents if AIDS was explained in a rational way. "Their strategy was, 'The *kids* will be the educational leaders,'" recalled Jill, who eventually decided to become a surgeon. "We will teach the students the facts, then they will teach the parents. This will defuse the situation right from the start."

Hamilton County school officials asked Ryan to wait for two weeks after classes resumed until he came to school. During those two weeks, students at Hamilton Heights would be educated about AIDS with a special series of classes, speakers, and assemblies. As student body president, Jill spoke at an assembly that emphasized the importance of tolerance. Her father, Jim, launched a separate community initiative. As a member of the local chapter in Cicero of Kiwanis International, he asked the service organization to launch a community education program about AIDS. Civic leaders and merchants attended breakfasts and other events that focused on appropriate responses to families with AIDS patients.

The Whites were heartened by the reactions to their arrival in Cicero. During the summer, though, Ryan's health became fragile. He vomited frequently and was tired constantly. When he was placed on various medications to help treat his AIDS symptoms, Ryan sometimes had frightening reactions. According to Jeanne, he endured "diabetic-like seizures" twice. Both times, the seizures subsided when his medications were altered.

Then Doctor Martin Kleiman prescribed AZT, a new drug that was proving to be effective for adult patients with AIDS. The drug seemed to help, but Ryan continued to look pale and gaunt. Because Jeanne had returned to work at Delco Electronics Corporation after a brief period at home to focus on her family, she periodically asked Jill to drive Ryan to his appointments with Kleiman. As a senior, Jill already had her driver's license. She and Ryan had long, profound talks in her Toyota en route to his appointments. "Ryan was very aware that he might die young, and he was at peace with that," Jill recalled. "Ryan wanted to live, though. It sounds contrived, but he knew he had a mission in life."

As August approached, residents of Indianapolis and surrounding communities became increasingly caught up in the excitement of hosting the Pan American Games, an international sporting event that would be the largest, multiday athletic competition in the history of the Hoosier capital. Athletes, coaches, and spectators were expected from Brazil, Cuba, Mexico, Canada, Argentina, Suriname, Jamaica, and other countries across the Western Hemisphere. Along with top American athletes, the international visitors planned to compete in sports ranging from basketball, track and field, and gymnastics to diving, swimming, baseball, and field hockey. Civic leaders considered the Pan Am Games to be a "coming out" celebration for Indianapolis on an international stage.

The Whites, along with thousands of people living in central Indiana, found themselves affected by the Pan Am Games. Andrea, who continued to roller skate occasionally even though she was not competing on a regular basis, was selected to be among the skating entertainers in a spectacular opening ceremony at the world-famous Indianapolis Motor Speedway. The Disney-produced opening ceremony featured fireworks, gymnasts, musicians, costumed mascots, and scores of other athletes and entertainers in a gala that was part lavish concert, part sporting showcase.

Sadly, Jeanne and Ryan missed Andrea's roller skating role at the Speedway. They were caught in a major traffic snarl en route

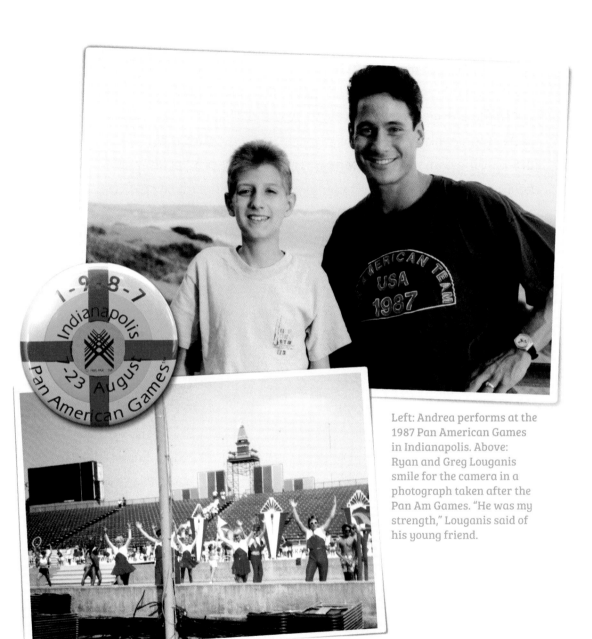

Left: Andrea performs at the 1987 Pan American Games in Indianapolis. Above: Ryan and Greg Louganis smile for the camera in a photograph taken after the Pan Am Games. "He was my strength," Louganis said of his young friend.

to the racetrack, where 80,000 people attended the opening ceremonies. It was yet another disappointment for Jeanne regarding Andrea's skating activities.

The Pan Am Games, though, put fifteen-year-old Ryan in the spotlight at the Indiana University Natatorium. Greg Louganis quickly became a superstar of the competition, achieving a record point total and becoming the first athlete in diving history to win both of the sport's gold medals (in springboard and platform diving) in three consecutive Pan Am Games. On the evening of his historic "triple double," as Louganis's feat was called, the aerial athlete draped a gold medal around Ryan's neck. Louganis handed his rose bouquet to Jeanne. "I've been putting these (medals) in a scrapbook," Ryan said, describing Louganis as one of his heroes. The diver, though, took the media opportunity to praise Ryan. "He's got a lot of strength, and he's very determined," Louganis said. "I have a lot of things to learn from him."

Jeanne reported that Ryan's health was improving thanks to the AZT. To spectators at the Natatorium, though, Ryan appeared feeble, pale, and underweight, particularly when he stood next to— and was photographed alongside—bronzed, muscular Louganis, who is of Samoan heritage.

As the Pan Am Games were winding down, Hamilton Heights High School began classes for the new school year. The two weeks of AIDS-focused instruction started. Faculty members wanted to make certain Ryan's arrival unfolded smoothly in many ways. Before he showed up at his freshman biology class, the teacher asked one of the most altruistic students, effervescent Heather McNew, if she would volunteer to be Ryan's lab partner. She immediately agreed.

"The first thing Ryan said to me was, 'Do you have a pencil?' because he had forgotten his," Heather recalled. "I said, 'Sure,' and handed him an extra pencil. He seemed so grateful for that simple gesture. Then, Ryan started making me laugh. We liked each other right away, and we ended up having all of our classes together. He definitely became my best friend."

Just as she had done for his medical appointments, Jill drove Ryan to school in the mornings in her Toyota. Often, crews from local and national television programs were waiting to film Ryan's arrival at Hamilton Heights, irritating him. According to Jill, the two friends frequently made a game of avoiding the media, sometimes by hiding in bushes before sneaking into the high school.

Occasionally, though, Ryan accepted an offer to be interviewed on camera, particularly if the program was targeted at teenagers or preteens. His biggest impact early on came when he was profiled on an episode of *3-2-1 Contact*, a syndicated, after-school television series that was nationally distributed. With a loyal audience of young viewers and a raft of Emmy Awards, *3-2-1 Contact* presented educational topics, including scientific issues, in captivating ways.

The episode focusing on Ryan was titled "I Have AIDS: A Teenager's Story." It opened with a close-up of Ryan staring directly into the camera. In his distinctly raspy voice, he introduced himself this way: "I'm Ryan White, I'm 16 years old, and I have AIDS." A narrator then elaborated for the audience of young viewers: "Ryan White is a pretty cool guy, probably like a lot of your friends. If Ryan White went to your school, what would you do? Would you be friends with him?"

The narrator went on to describe the controversy about Ryan's

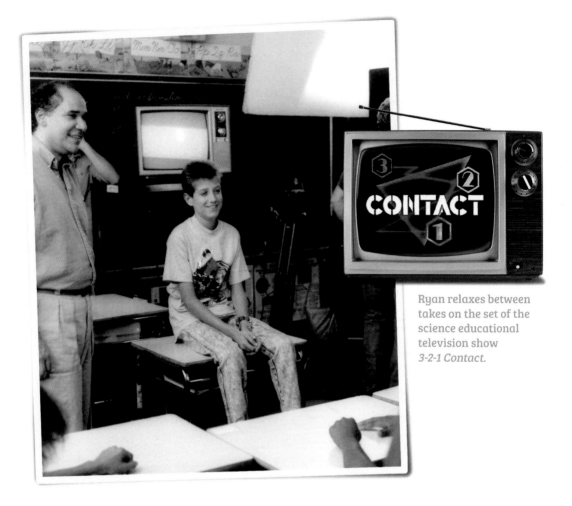

Ryan relaxes between takes on the set of the science educational television show *3-2-1 Contact.*

school attendance in the Kokomo area, then mentioned the AIDS education sessions during the first two weeks of classes at Hamilton Heights. Sequences in the *3-2-1 Contact* episode included footage of Ryan riding his bicycle in his new neighborhood and playfully interacting with Jeanne.

In addition to attending classes with Heather, Ryan talked with her on the phone almost every evening. The two also helped each other with their homework. "We were opposites, but ideal for each other," she recalled. "I was good in English, but not in math. Ryan was good in math, but not in English."

Before the *3-2-1 Contact* episode was shown across the country, Ryan even landed a job. When he was traveling from Kokomo and Cicero to Kleiman's office near downtown Indianapolis for various treatments, Ryan had noticed the bustling Castleton area on the north side of the Hoosier capital. Among the long rows of retail outlets, he was intrigued by Maui Surf and Sport, a skateboard shop. Ryan continually asked his mom to stop at Maui so he could buy skateboarder outfits, mirrored sunglasses, and magazines about skateboarding. (He considered skateboarding to be an ideal passion until he could earn his driver's license and slide behind the wheel of a car.) After Ryan turned sixteen years old in December 1987, Maui's owner offered Ryan a part-time job. He was delighted. Ryan's duties primarily involved assembling skateboards. Customers, though, began dropping by the shop just to meet him.

Also a few weeks after Ryan's sixteenth birthday, Indiana governor Robert Orr and other state officials, including Myers, came to Hamilton Heights to honor Ryan and his classmates. At a ceremony in the school's gym, Ryan was named a Sagamore of the Wabash, at that time one of the top awards given by an Indiana governor. All of the other students at the high school (nearly six hundred teenagers) received a special award called "Spirit of the Heartland" for welcoming and accepting Ryan. The award consisted of a lapel pin depicting a handshake and the name of the newly created honor. "Instead of dissolving into a scared pack, this community came together," Orr said. "You took on one of the most difficult questions of our time."

Later that evening, ABC News named Ryan as "Person of the Week." Peter Jennings, the anchorman of *ABC Evening News*, announced Ryan was chosen because of his inspirational attitude and the bravery of his crusade to attend school. Ryan, the anchorman told the national television audience, was helping lessen hostility and unfair reactions to people living with AIDS.

The national attention meant people as far away as California wanted to meet Ryan. Athletes and Entertainers for Kids, a nonprofit organization of sports stars and other celebrities, invited him to Los Angeles to help launch a new national program. The group sponsored school visits by athletes to meet at-risk children as well as celebrity visits to hospitals for talks with young patients. Athletes and Entertainers for Kids was planning a new program of school presentations. Celebrities were preparing to visit schools to talk about AIDS with young people. Athletes and Entertainers for Kids asked the Whites to come to Los Angeles to promote the launch of the national program.

Ryan accepted the invitation. For the trip to Southern California, he not only was accompanied by Jeanne and Andrea, but also by Heather. He asked his classmate to go with them because, he explained, he wanted to have a "date" by his side at parties attended by former basketball superstar Kareem Abdul-Jabbar, television actress Alyssa Milano, and other famous Americans. "I felt like a princess," Heather recalled. "Ryan was getting used to these kinds of events, so I just tried to follow his lead in remaining calm."

Lou Ann Baker, the AIDS education coordinator for Indiana, said she was continually impressed by Ryan's attitude. "Unlike the way many teenagers react if they are chosen to meet celebrities, he never bragged," she said. "It was part of his approach of, "I'm going to be a typical kid.'"

Next, though, came the most intimidating, and important, invitation of all. Considering that the invitation came from some of the most powerful people in Washington D.C., Ryan felt compelled to accept it. The Presidential Commission on AIDS wanted Ryan to come to the nation's capital. The commission, which met on Capitol Hill, also wanted to hear from Jill as Hamilton Heights' student body president. That meant teenagers Ryan and Jill would be making presentations to members of the cabinet and the U.S. Congress.

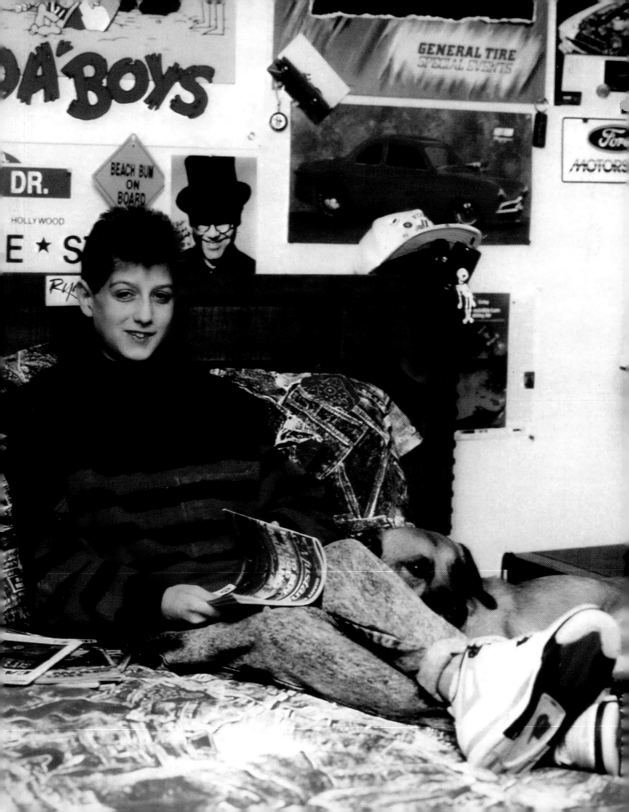

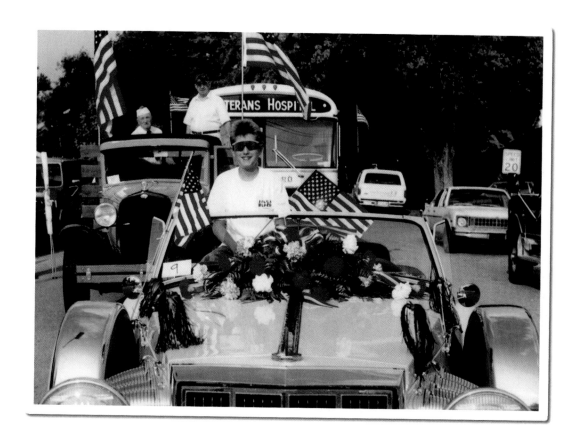

"I never wanted to be famous.
It's embarrassing to be famous for
being sick, especially with a disease
like AIDS. I never wanted to be the
'AIDS boy' who was always in the
news. I just wanted to be like
every other kid my age."

"To tell you the truth, AIDS didn't seem like such a big deal at first—just another illness. I'd been sick with an incurable disease since the day I was born, and I was used to it."

7

In his Washington, D.C., hotel room, Ryan White did not want to get out of bed. He was dreading another public appearance. This one in early March 1988 involved extra stress because it would be on Capitol Hill, speaking to the President's Commission on AIDS. The panel included members of the U.S. Congress from across the country as well as cabinet members, such as Surgeon General Everett Koop, a pediatric surgeon.

The political and medical leaders wanted to hear about prejudice toward people with AIDS from the sixteen-year-old boy whose crusade to attend school in Indiana had captured their attention. They also wanted to hear from Jill Stewart, Hamilton Heights High School's student body president, about how and why her classmates welcomed Ryan with minimal controversy and hostility.

During the day before their appearance at the AIDS commission, Ryan, Jeanne, and Jill visited national monuments and other landmarks in Washington, including the Vietnam War Memorial. Then, all three of them were interviewed on ABC's *Nightline* by the news show's host, Ted Koppel.

On the morning of March 3, a Thursday, Ryan resisted getting out of bed. He seldom enjoyed public speaking, even though once he forced himself to step behind a microphone, he invariably, as Jill put it, "nailed" his talks. Because the presentation to the AIDS commission involved such an influential audience and would be covered by television networks and other media, Jill chose to wear one of her best dresses and pearls.

Ryan took the opposite approach. After he was dragged out of bed by Jeanne, Ryan decided to, as he phrased it in his autobiography, put on "what I'd wear to school." That meant jeans, a comfortable shirt, and his favorite sneakers. They were high tops, and he left the laces untied as he walked across Capitol Hill.

Before the AIDS commission, Ryan and Jill sat at a spare, wooden table with microphones. The U.S. Congress members and other commissioners faced them from behind a long desk mounted on a stage. Rows of photographers and cameramen crouched below the desk with their equipment, clicking and whirring. "I came face to face with death at 13 years old," Ryan said, referring to his AIDS diagnosis. He told the commissioners that he refused to capitulate to the diagnosis and decided instead "to live a normal life, to go to school, be with my friends, and enjoy day-to-day activties."

Despite some brief fits of coughing during his presentation, Ryan, as usual, came off well. He described the challenges the Whites had confronted in Howard County. "I was labeled a troublemaker, my mom an unfit mother, and I was not welcome anywhere. People would get up and leave so they would not have to sit anywhere near me. Even at church, people would not shake my hand," he said. After moving to Cicero, daily life changed, Ryan continued. He emphasized he felt accepted at Hamilton Heights and looked forward to graduating as a member of the Class of 1991.

Then it was Jill's turn at the microphone. She described the AIDS education program at Hamilton Heights. She also emphasized that her classmates had benefited from Ryan's presence and from witnessing his courage in confronting a fatal disorder. "He puts life in perspective," she said. "These things you can't measure."

Back in Indiana, Jill had come to regard Doctor Martin Kleiman, the infectious disease specialist who was treating Ryan at Riley Hospital, as a role model. After observing his interactions with Ryan when Jill drove her friend to appointments, she decided to become a physician herself.

Unfortunately, Ryan needed to see Kleiman much more frequently now. He often was sick, sometimes with various infections, sometimes with fevers, and other times with stomach distress that caused him to vomit almost anything he ate. "He really was chronically ill," Kleiman recalled. "The AIDS was progressive. Ryan was brave, though. He was unaffected by the media attention. He was very down-to-earth and bright—not in an educated way, but in terms of having excellent judgment."

The public was generally unaware of Ryan's continual, serious health struggles. In part that was because, as Jeanne noted, he only agreed to media appearances if he looked at least somewhat healthy. "At that point, most people with AIDS who were on TV were about to die," she recalled. "Ryan wanted to show you could live with AIDS." Even friends sometimes couldn't tell when Ryan was ill. "He wasn't a complainer," Jill said. "Sometimes you'd only know he was in pain because he'd get quiet."

Ryan was well enough to accept an invitation that seemed particularly intriguing. Joining the other celebrities who had extended support to Ryan, pop superstar Michael Jackson invited the Whites to spend a day at his Neverland Ranch in Southern California. Located on more than 2,500 acres, Neverland Ranch was known to have a zoo, a movie theater, an arcade of video games, lavish gardens, a swimming pool, and an amusement park with bumper cars and a Ferris wheel. Ryan, Jeanne, and Andrea accepted the offer.

During their visit, Jackson gave the Whites a tour of the secluded ranch and of his sprawling mansion. Although the family's initial stay was just for one day, the legendary pop star apparently paid close attention to his guests. He noticed that Ryan, who by now had his driver's license, carried a copy of *Mustang Monthly*, one of his favorite car magazines. When the Whites returned to Indiana, they were notified by a local auto dealership that Jackson had purchased a red Mustang for Ryan. As soon as the flashy car was delivered to the Whites' home, the Mustang became Ryan's passion. He regularly asked his best friend, Heather McNew, to join him in "cruising."

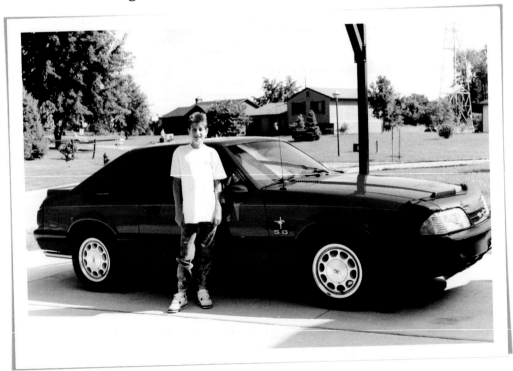

She would meet Ryan at a strip shopping center in Cicero and slide into his Mustang. If the weather was warm, Ryan would lower the car's sun roof as he drove in a long loop north to the town of Tipton, then back down to Cicero. They often cruised for three hours, night after night, according to Heather. "He was a crazy driver," she recalled, smiling. "But what would you expect? He was a teenager with a brand new, red Mustang. We'd have the music on. It's amazing how much pure joy we got out of this."

Thanks to the eye-catching car, Ryan also met a neighbor in Cicero who eventually would play an important role with the White family. The neighbor, Roy Ginder, was a single father of young children. He worked as a mechanic at a body shop in nearby Carmel. Roy, who owned a rebuilt 1957 Chevrolet, noticed Ryan in his driveway, trying to tinker with his new Mustang. Roy offered to help Ryan customize the car with adjustments and enhancements. The two developed a bond. Without telling Jeanne, they even drag raced (Roy in his Chevy versus Ryan in his Mustang) near Cicero in a secluded area.

Although the drag racing was a secret, Ryan was leading an increasingly public life. In May, *People* magazine featured him on its cover. Titled "Amazing Grace," the six-page article hailed Ryan for exuding "a great gift for living." Photographs in the popular, nationally distributed magazine included a candid picture of Ryan skateboarding in Cicero while walking his dog, Wally, on a long leash. Another photo depicted Ryan during his Disneyland trip with Elton John, who posed in an oversized wig, a jazzy tuxedo, and elongated sunglasses. The *People* article also featured photos of Ryan with diver Greg Louganis at the Indiana University

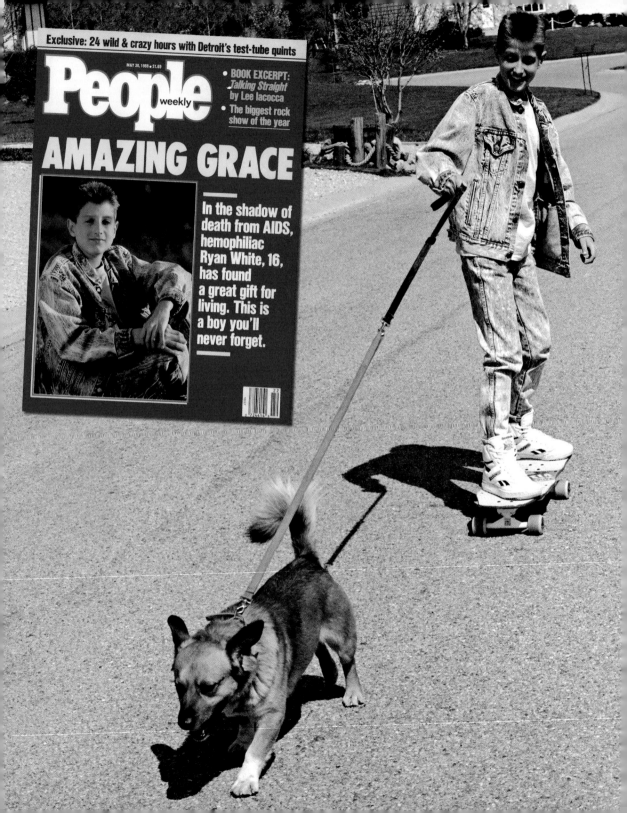

Natatorium, and with Heather in his algebra class at Hamilton Heights.

At school, Ryan and Heather joined the yearbook staff. Heather also was a cross-country star at Hamilton Heights, even setting a school record in the mile. Ryan enjoyed attending her meets and cheering her on. "He became my biggest fan," Heather recalled. The two soon were inseparable.

When Jackson extended a follow-up invitation to the Whites in June to visit Neverland Ranch, Ryan asked Heather to accompany the family. She instantly agreed. During the visit, Jackson taught Heather how to ride a specialized, four-wheeled scooter that resembled a dirt bike. The group also visited the zoo on the Neverland compound. In addition to admiring giraffes and other exotic animals, Ryan and Heather met Jackson's pet monkeys, which had drawn national attention. "They were well-behaved, and they were wearing T-shirts and other 'people' clothes," Heather recalled.

When the group encountered the monkeys, the pets were disembarking from a chauffeured car. Ryan and Heather were told the monkeys were returning from an etiquette class in which Jackson had enrolled them. "I realize the situation seems weird to many people, but I happen to love monkeys, and it didn't seem weird to me," Heather recalled years later. "Also, I didn't notice any weird behavior from Michael Jackson."

During the California trip, Ryan appeared at a tribute organized by Athletes and Entertainers for Kids to honor basketball sensation Kareem Abdul-Jabbar, who was retiring after a long career playing for the Milwaukee Bucks and the Los Angeles Lakers. During the tribute, which was televised, Ryan stood beside Abdul-Jabbar, who

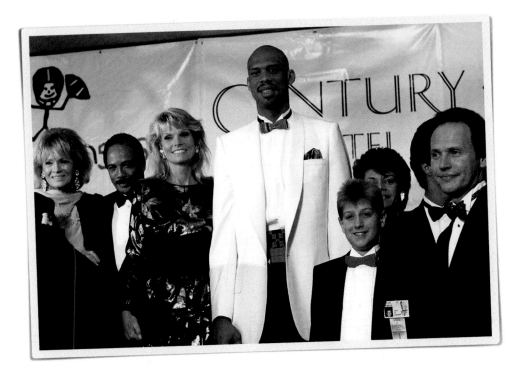

is seven feet, two inches tall. The contrast between the two was even starker than the one between Ryan and Louganis.

While the Whites were in Southern California, Athletes and Entertainers for Kids also arranged for Ryan to join several teenage television stars at Disneyland for the grand opening of a ride that's become wildly popular since then: Splash Mountain.

Other out-of-state trips for Ryan were focused primarily on presentations about coping with AIDS. In May he spoke at Boys Town in Omaha, Nebraska. During the event at a concert hall attended by hundreds of students, teachers, ministers, and parents, some of the students, many of whom were about Ryan's age, asked blunt questions. "How does it feel knowing you're going to die?" one boy wanted to know. Ryan responded, "Someday you'll die too . . . It's how you live your life that counts."

Another boy wondered if he was frightened to die. "No," Ryan replied. "If I were worried about dying, I'd die. I'm not afraid. I'm just not ready yet,"

More speaking requests followed, several from even larger audiences at some of the most famous venues in the country. In July Ryan traveled to New Orleans for a convention of the National Education Association. At the Superdome sports stadium, Ryan spoke to 10,000 teachers who gathered for the convention. The teachers gave him a standing ovation. Also during the summer, the Whites traveled to North Carolina for the filming of *The Ryan White Story*. Weeks earlier, the director of the television-movie had visited Cicero, where Ryan treated him to a cruise in the Mustang, and terrified him with his speeding. Even so, the two developed a bond. For the filming in Statesville, North Carolina, the Whites were asked to be on the set almost continually to ensure accuracy.

Ryan also was invited to play the small role of "Chad," a young AIDS patient whom Ryan encounters during one of his hospitalizations. (Ryan himself was portrayed by Lukas Haas, a young actor who had won rave reviews three years earlier for his role in the hit movie *Witness*.) Jeanne, in turn, developed a close friendship with the actress chosen to portray her, televison star Judith Light. Small roles in the movie were played by Charles Vaughan Sr., the White family's attorney, and other friends who visited the set.

During the filming in August, Ryan's health was almost consistently good despite long hours on the set. He ended up enjoying the experience and even ran errands for the crew, securing the job title of "second assistant director." He had high hopes for the production. "If enough people saw it, maybe other kids with

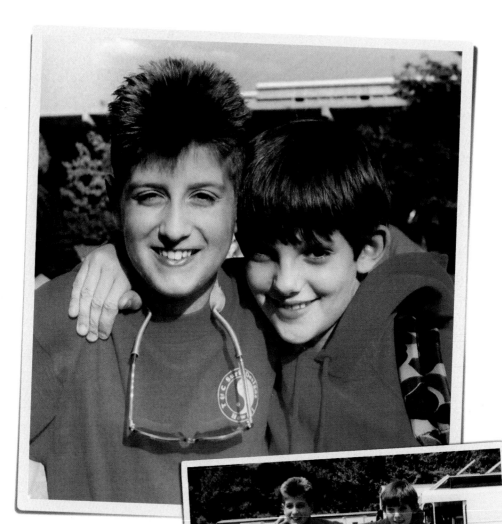

Ryan and Lukas Haas, the star of the television-movie *The Ryan White Story* that aired on the ABC network on January 16, 1989. Haas had won fame years before by playing a young Amish boy who witnesses a murder in the Harrison Ford film *Witness* (1985).

AIDS I'd never know, would be treated better," he wrote in his autobiography. Ryan added that his responsibilities on the set were enlightening: "Now I knew I was good at something besides being sick."

Ryan began accepting more speaking invitations. They included an offer from television personality Phil Donahue, the host of one of the most popular afternoon talk shows in the country. *Donahue* was taped before a studio audience that joined the host in questioning his guest. For the show with Ryan, Donahue's audience was filled with teenagers, enabling Ryan to share insights "kid-to-kid." Once again, he was a media hit.

Just before the start of the 1989–90 school year, though, Ryan began struggling with an array of medical setbacks. He had looked forward to classes at Hamilton Heights, but his absences became frequent. Even when Ryan showed up, he usually attended school for just four hours. "Very often, he'd wake up full of energy in the morning, take his shower, get dressed, eat a bite of breakfast—and then be too exhausted to go to school," Jeanne later noted in her autobiography.

Ryan's health issues ranged from severe chills and fevers to increasingly worse liver dysfunctions. He also suffered from a hernia, a torn muscle that occurred after bouts of deep, painful coughing. The hernia caused intense pain when Ryan sat or walked. With an otherwise healthy patient, the hernia could have been surgically removed. Kleiman, however, concluded Ryan should not undergo surgery. Because of the progression of AIDS and Ryan's other medical challenges, an operation was deemed too risky. That conclusion not only alarmed Jeanne, it distressed Ryan. He was beginning to realize he might not have many more, if any, rebounds.

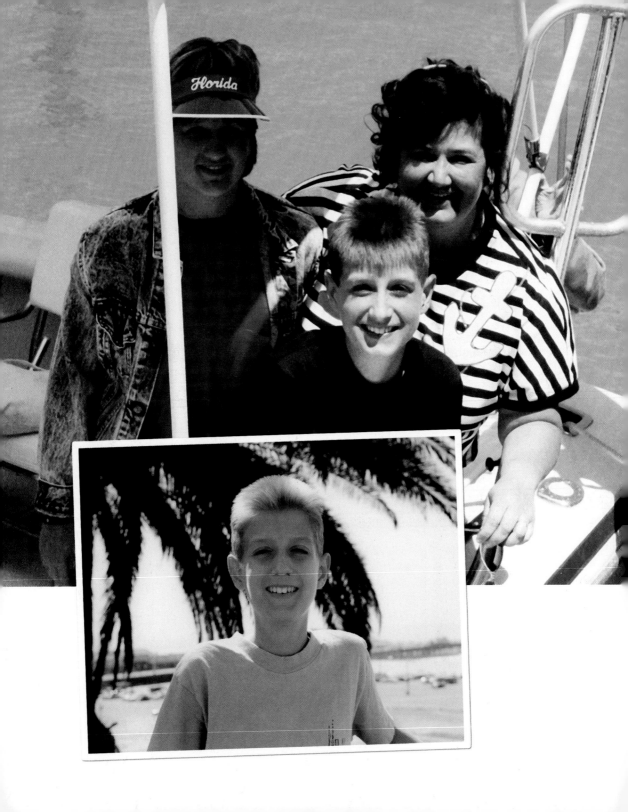

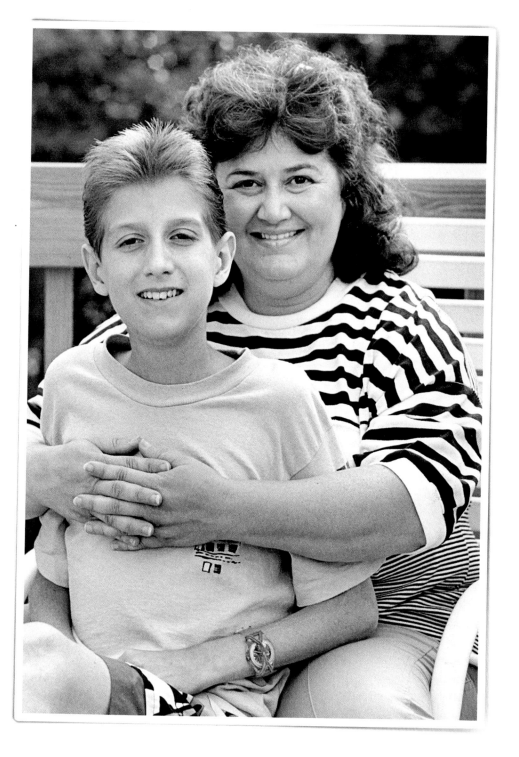

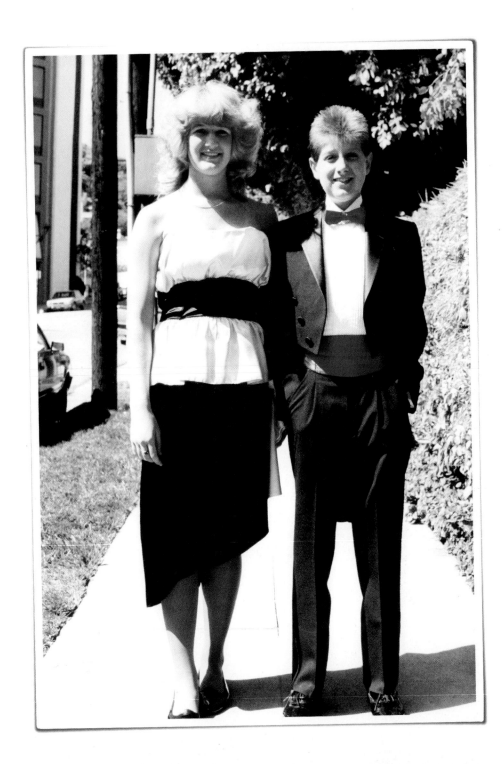

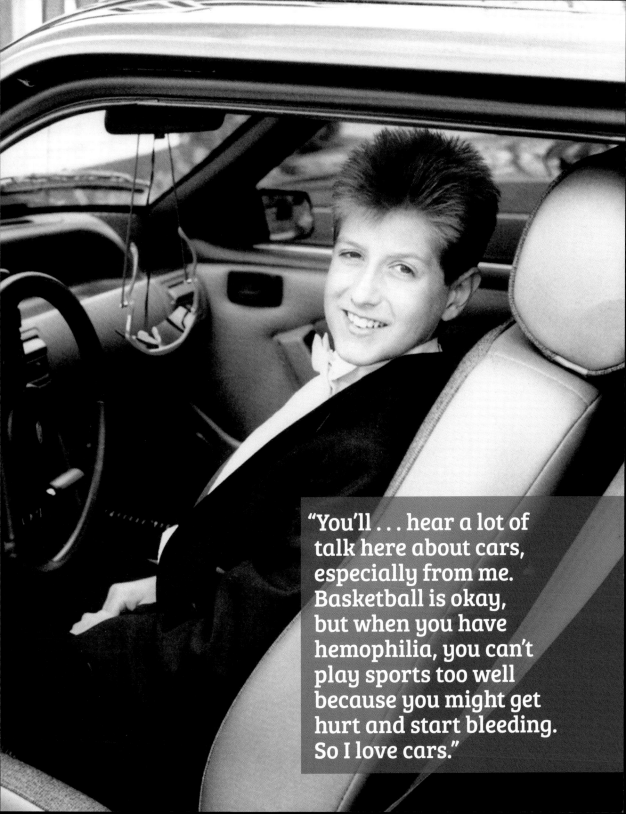

"You'll . . . hear a lot of talk here about cars, especially from me. Basketball is okay, but when you have hemophilia, you can't play sports too well because you might get hurt and start bleeding. So I love cars."

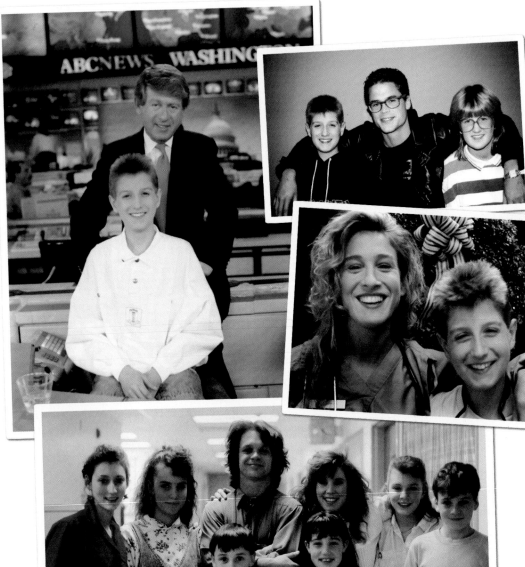
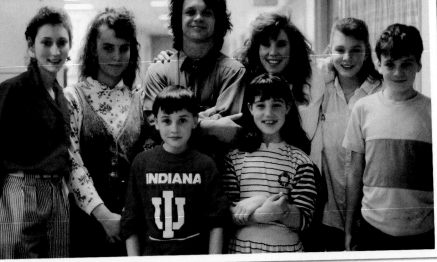

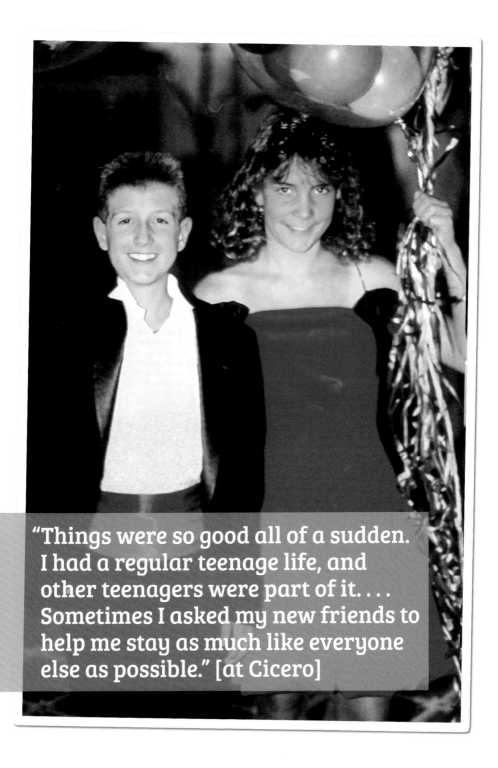

"Things were so good all of a sudden. I had a regular teenage life, and other teenagers were part of it. . . . Sometimes I asked my new friends to help me stay as much like everyone else as possible." [at Cicero]

"When I breathed, I rattled. Sometimes I ran out of breath completely. In the middle of a conversation, I'd have to stop talking, rest my head on my hands, and take some short pants."

8

In spite of his various health challenges, Ryan White was able to tape some radio and television public-service announcements about AIDS. The first, broadcast on World AIDS Day in November 1989, was targeted at teenagers and other young people. He opened the announcement this way: "Hello, I'm Ryan White. You know, as much as we've talked to you about AIDS, a lot of you still aren't listening. Today is World AIDS Day, so please listen." Ryan then discussed the ways AIDS is transmitted and urged young people to resist pressure to try drugs or sex.

At Hamilton Heights High School, Ryan kept up with his work on the yearbook staff. Heather McNew was a copy editor; Ryan assisted with copy editing and helped in various other ways. He also volunteered to assist one of Hamilton Height's science teachers. His absences from school, however, increased dramatically. In early December, Ryan turned eighteen, normally a cause for celebration among teenagers. But his health had become fragile. AIDS was leaving him vulnerable to a series of infections. Even his hearing was affected. On some days, Ryan barely could understand what people were saying. He also suffered from constant, unrelenting chills.

During the break for the holidays, Ryan received another invitation from Michael Jackson to visit Neverland Ranch. In his autobiography, Ryan quoted the pop singer as telling him on the phone: "We've got to get together and goof off again." Before Jeanne allowed Ryan to travel to California, she consulted with Doctor Martin Kleiman to make certain the trip would not jeopardize his health. After receiving assurances that medical personnel could respond quickly to an emergency at the isolated ranch, Kleiman agreed to the trip to Neverland.

So in late December, after Ryan celebrated Christmas with his family in Cicero, he flew to Los Angeles. He brought an electrical heater and wore a leather coat even in the California sun.

At the Los Angeles airport, he was met by Jackson's security guards and a limousine. During the three-hour ride to Neverland Ranch, Ryan suffered from cramps and a stomach ache. He continued to feel ill even after he settled into his bungalow at the ranch. (The Neverland compound included several bungalows for guests.) From his cottage, Ryan phoned Jeanne and wondered whether he should have made the trip.

But he perked up after savoring a hearty dinner with Jackson. According to Ryan's autobiography, the two then enjoyed a movie marathon in the private theater at Neverland. They watched a series of movies featuring the Three Stooges slapstick comedy team.

The next morning, Ryan joined Jackson on a shopping spree for toys that the pop singer intended to donate to children. During a later shopping trip, one of Jackson's staff members bought a bomber jacket for Ryan because the singer thought his friend needed a heavier coat. Jackson also gave him a new stereo system before Ryan returned to Indiana on New Year's Day.

Unfortunately Ryan's health worsened at the beginning of 1990. Because of his hernia and a perpetually swollen stomach,

Ryan often slouched when he walked. He coughed constantly in the Indiana winter weather. His legs became pocked with sores; every day, Jeanne placed fresh bandages on them. Not only did Ryan stay home from school, he also rarely even had the stamina to tackle home-instruction assignments from his teachers. Whenever possible, Ryan would rev up the energy to polish his red Mustang. Sometimes that would exhaust him for the rest of the day.

To bolster Ryan's strength, Kleiman instructed him to consume a protein-laden drink several times daily. Ryan hated the drink's taste and texture. Attempting to make the concoction more appealing, Jeanne mixed it with orange juice or milk. Nothing helped much, in Ryan's opinion. He continued to describe it as "horrible." In February, though, he was strong enough to return to Hamilton Heights. Ryan even received permission from Kleiman to take another trip to Southern California. Athletes and Entertainers for Kids had extended an enticing invitation. The organization wanted Ryan to present a public-service award to President Ronald Reagan at an elegant party.

All of this energized Ryan like a shot in the arm, and he started making long-range plans again. Ryan asked Heather McNew to go with him to Hamilton Heights' prom, which was scheduled for April 28. The two went clothes shopping, and Ryan expressed his preference that she wear an "emerald green" dress on their big night.

Just before Ryan, Jeanne, and Andrea left for California in March, though, various health problems returned. He suffered from fevers that kept him up at night. His hernia continued to bother him. Ryan also struggled with prolonged coughing fits. Health issues persisted in the California sun and at the lavish parties. The event with President Ronald Reagan and First Lady Nancy Reagan was billed as an "Oscar Party" because it occurred on the same evening as the Academy Awards ceremony.

The setting was the posh Beverly Wilshire Hotel. In addition to the Reagans, dozens of television stars attended the gala. Although Ryan tried to come across as carefree, he was noticeably frail and lethargic. Nancy Reagan quickly grabbed his hand and clasped it for most of the party. "She whispered to me, 'He's not doing well—I can tell,'" Jeanne recalled.

At another party, Ryan appeared with a celebrity affiliated with Athletes and Entertainers for Kids who had long offered support to the Whites: professional football star Howie Long of the Los Angeles Raiders. Kareem Abdul-Jabbar joined them at the gala as well. Ryan was feeling so sick, though, that he asked permission to leave early.

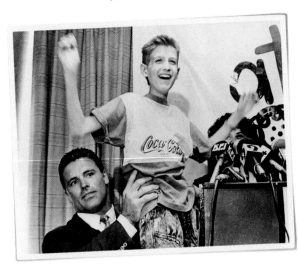

Football star Howie Long of the Oakland Raiders holds Ryan up during a press conference for an Athletes and Entertainers for Kids benefit in California.

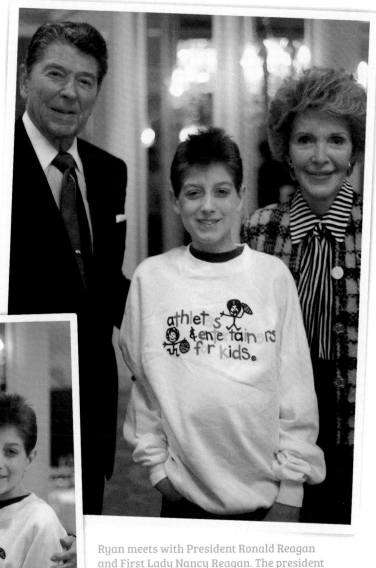

Ryan meets with President Ronald Reagan and First Lady Nancy Reagan. The president noted that "Ryan White touched our lives in a special way. His ready smile, his youthful innocence, his simple desire to just live his life tugged at our hearts in a way we will always remember. How we wanted to hug him and make him better."

Back at the Whites' hotel, Ryan crawled into bed. He spent the next day sleeping. After coughing fits returned, Ryan finally confided to Jeanne that they needed to fly back to Indianapolis so he could be examined by Kleiman.

Alarmed, Jeanne made arrangements for them to return aboard the next available flight on March 29. It was an overnight flight with few other passengers, enabling Ryan to stretch out across several seats. After the plane landed, Jeanne immediately checked him into Riley Hospital for Children. Kleiman concluded that Ryan was suffering from a severe respiratory infection.

From the hospital, Ryan made a phone call to Gloria Hale, his grandmother, who was in Florida. He tried to sound upbeat, but she was alarmed by his weak voice and frequent gasps. After their talk, Ryan struggled so much with each breath that he could not make more telephone calls. He was placed on oxygen. His condition rapidly deteriorated. He was moved to intensive care. To help Ryan breathe, Kleiman had him placed on a ventilator. Because the tube extended through his nose and mouth, he had to write notes to communicate with Jeanne. At his bedside, she began to pray. Ryan slipped into unconsciousness.

During the next week, word spread that Ryan was hospitalized at Riley and possibly near death. On April 2 hospital officials made a public announcement that Ryan was in critical condition in the intensive care unit. They said family members had requested no additional details about his condition be released.

Even so, the hospital was inundated with phone calls, cards, and letters from across the country. At his room in the intensive care unit, Jeanne and Andrea kept a bedside vigil. They were joined by Ryan's grandparents, who had flown up from Florida, and by friends such as Heather and Jill Stewart.

Elton John immediately made arrangements to fly to Indianapolis when he heard the grim news about Ryan. The rock star arrived with his security guards, whom he assigned to protect Jeanne and Andrea. "Elton John was totally sincere," Heather recalled. "He did whatever Jeanne needed, including answering the phone." He also visited other young patients in intensive care at Riley. Hoping that music might soothe or inspire Ryan, who remained unconscious, John brought a stereo into the room and played tapes of Jackson's hits.

Then, Jackson himself called the hospital. The phone receiver was cradled next to Ryan's ear so Jackson could urge him to get well. Sadly, no flickers from Ryan indicated he was aware of his famous friend's pleas.

Still hoping for a recovery, his friends and family kept talking to Ryan. They tried to coax him to respond with a smile or some other movement. Heather reminded Ryan about their date to go to the prom at the end of the month. John decorated Ryan's hospital room with banners sent by schoolchildren from across the country so there would be a festive touch amid the tubes, monitoring equipment, and other machines if Ryan regained consciousness. Nothing could help, however. Ryan did not come out of the coma. His blood pressure plummeted to levels that were alarmingly low. Kleiman indicated to Jeanne that Ryan was nearing the end. He was placed on a life-support system.

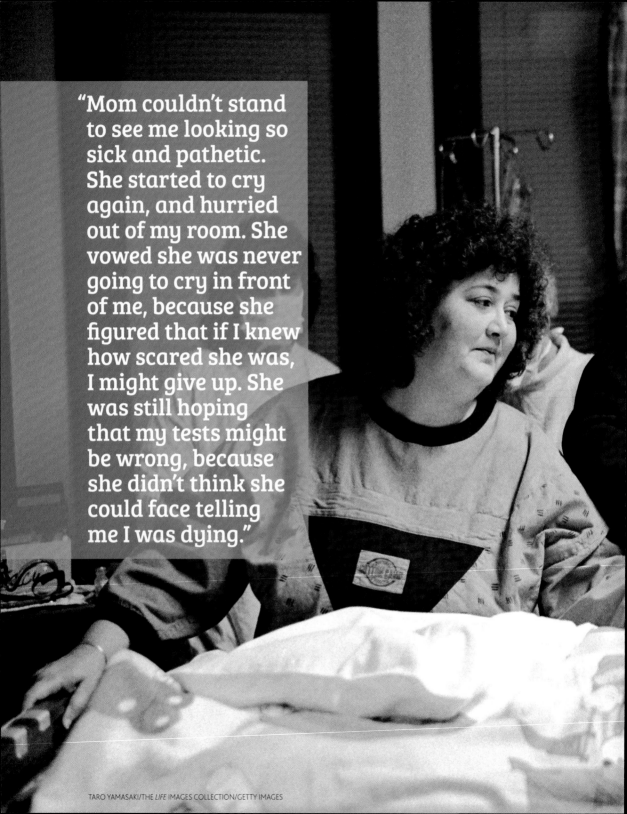

"Mom couldn't stand to see me looking so sick and pathetic. She started to cry again, and hurried out of my room. She vowed she was never going to cry in front of me, because she figured that if I knew how scared she was, I might give up. She was still hoping that my tests might be wrong, because she didn't think she could face telling me I was dying."

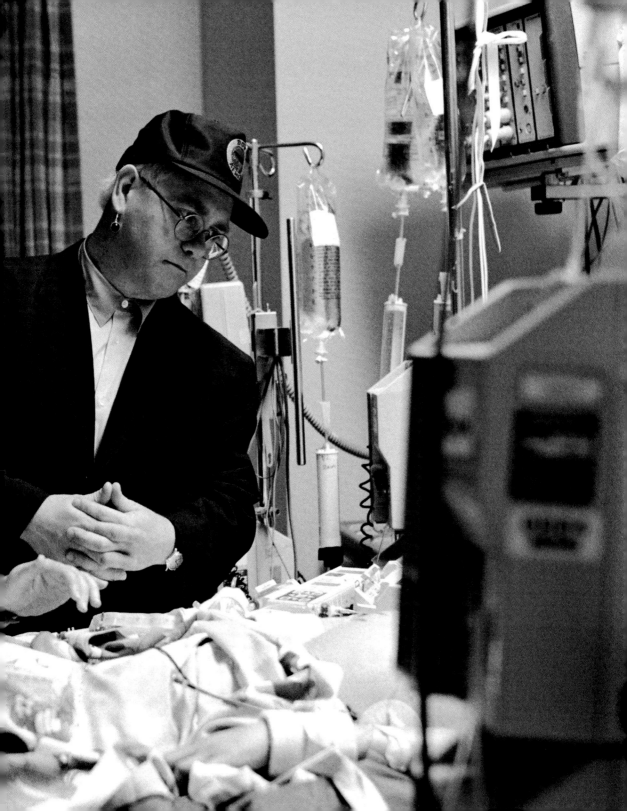

More friends began to arrive in Indianapolis, including famous supporters such as Phil Donahue. He joined John in making arrangements for Ryan's memorial service.

On the evening of April 7, a Saturday night, John left Ryan's bedside to make a cameo appearance at a massive concert at the nearby Hoosier Dome, the football stadium of the Indianapolis Colts; the concert was a fund-raiser to help the nation's struggling farmers. Organized by Indiana-born rock star John Mellencamp, Farm Aid IV was the fourth in a series of concerts for farm relief.

As a break from their long, exhausting days at the hospital, Andrea and Heather attended the concert to cheer on John. Announcing he was dedicating his performance to his friend Ryan, whose precarious condition was public knowledge by then, John sang "Candle in the Wind" to an overwhelming, heart-breaking response. "I looked into the crowd, and people were holding up their lighters, thousands of little vigils flickering in the darkness for my dying friend," John recalled in his memoir.

At the hospital, press conferences with updates about Ryan's condition were held twice daily. Carrie Jackson Van Dyke, a former television news anchor in Indianapolis who had befriended the Whites, spoke on behalf of the family. That way, Jeanne could remain by Ryan's bedside.

Finally, in the early hours of April 8, nurses flicked the lights in Ryan's room to see if he would react. When he did not respond, Jeanne leaned next to him and whispered that he could "let go." Ryan died shortly after 7 a.m. that day, which was Palm Sunday; he was just eighteen years old. Ryan had lived with his AIDS diagnosis for more than five years, nearly one-third of his life. In many ways, Riley Hospital had become a second home.

As soon as Ryan died at the hospital, his grieving family and close friends gathered in a circle there. The group included Jeanne; Andrea; Ryan's grandparents, Tom and Gloria Hale; Heather; and John. They said good-bye to Ryan and prayed for him.

News of Ryan's death spread quickly. Almost immediately, people ranging from neighbors and Hamilton Heights classmates to celebrities, journalists, curiosity seekers, and mourning strangers hurried to the Whites' house in Cicero on the chilly Sunday morning. They left flowers, cards, and gifts in the front lawn next to Ryan's cherished Mustang. The shiny red gift from Jackson was wheeled to the grass to serve as a makeshift memorial. By late morning, even Jackson had showed up at the Cicero house. Wearing a fedora, sunglasses, and a long, dark overcoat, the pop icon was accompanied by business tycoon Donald Trump, who had not been associated with Ryan's crusade to attend school.

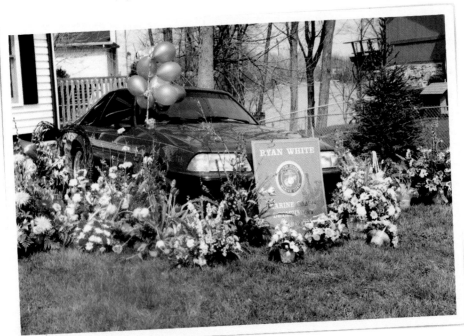

There was an explanation for Trump's presence. Jackson had been in Atlantic City, New Jersey, to visit Trump's new resort hotel and casino, the Taj Mahal, when they learned about Ryan's death. Trump immediately offered Jackson the use of his private jet; the pop singer then asked the business tycoon to accompany him to Indiana. Traveling with an entourage that included bodyguards and a chauffeur, neither celebrity spoke to the array of television and newspaper reporters who gathered in the Whites' front yard. The crowd also included autograph seekers and Hoosiers with video cameras as well as Cicero residents.

Several of Ryan's classmates came directly from Sunday church services, where they had been told the tragic news. At some churches, ministers even mentioned it from the pulpit. "I hope my kids grow up to be like Ryan, honest and decent," said Roy Ginder. Roy's son, Steve, who was twelve, pointed to his white sneakers. "Ryan gave me these," he said quietly. "He also gave my brother tennis shoes."

Along with other friends and classmates, they wanted to stress Ryan's generosity. They also had other reasons for talking about his fondness for things like high-top sneakers and fast cars. They wanted to reinforce something Ryan strived to emphasize most of his life, even when he was speaking from a podium in a massive stadium or being interviewed by a famous television personality: In so many ways, he always was a typical kid.

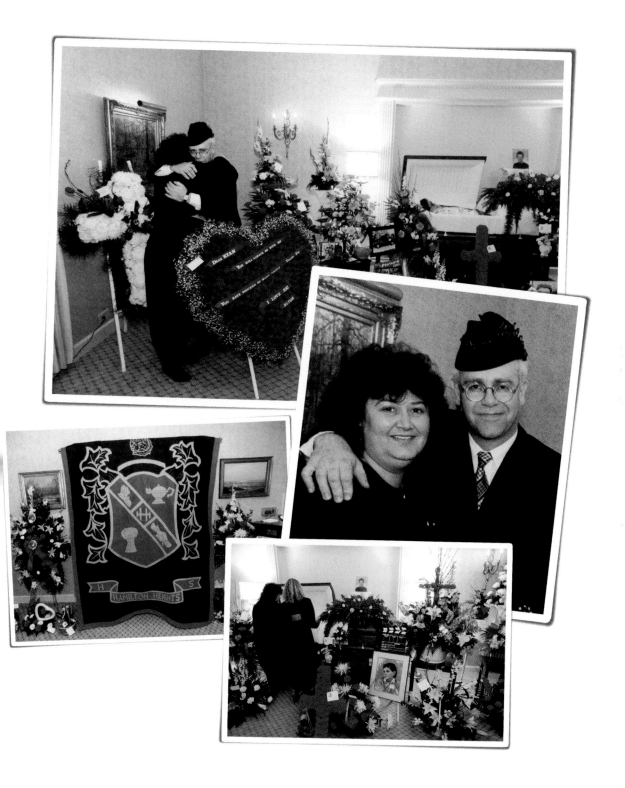

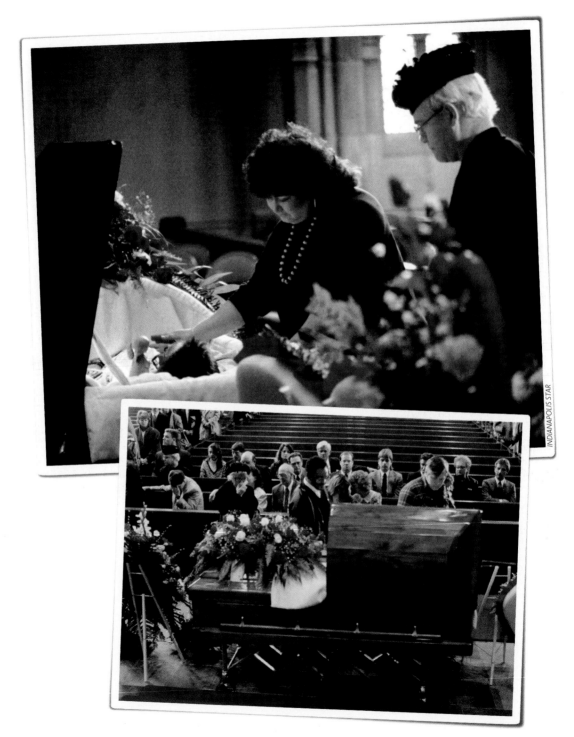

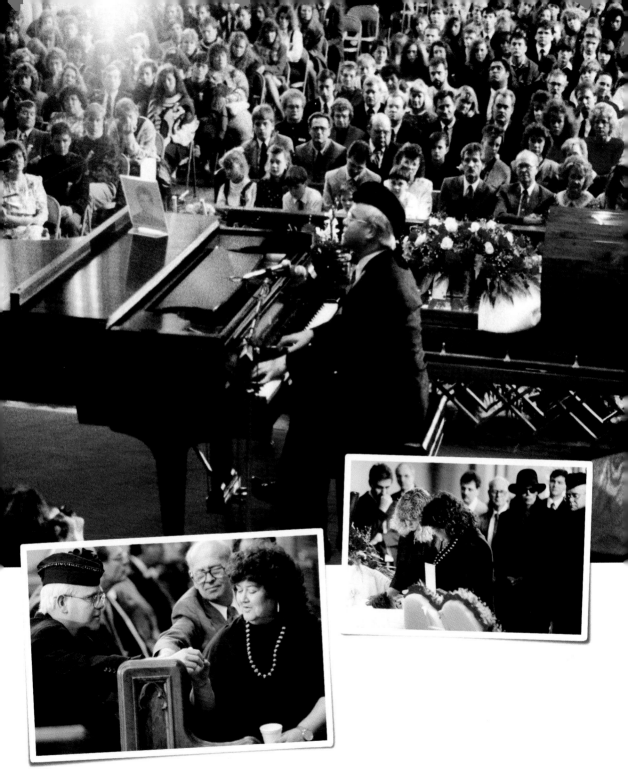

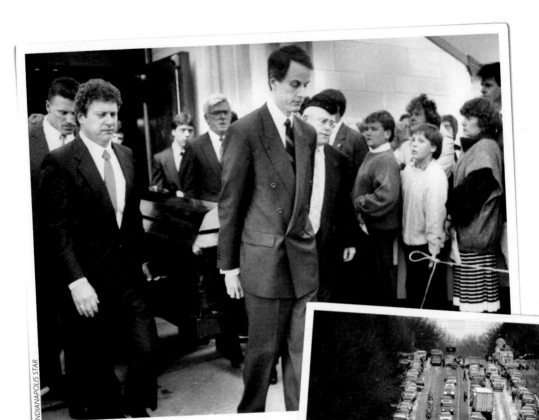

More than 1,500 friends and admirers attended Ryan's funeral. Serving as pallbearers were celebrities Elton John, Howie Long, Phil Donahue, and Ryan's friends Tommy Hale, Leo Joseph, and John Huffman.

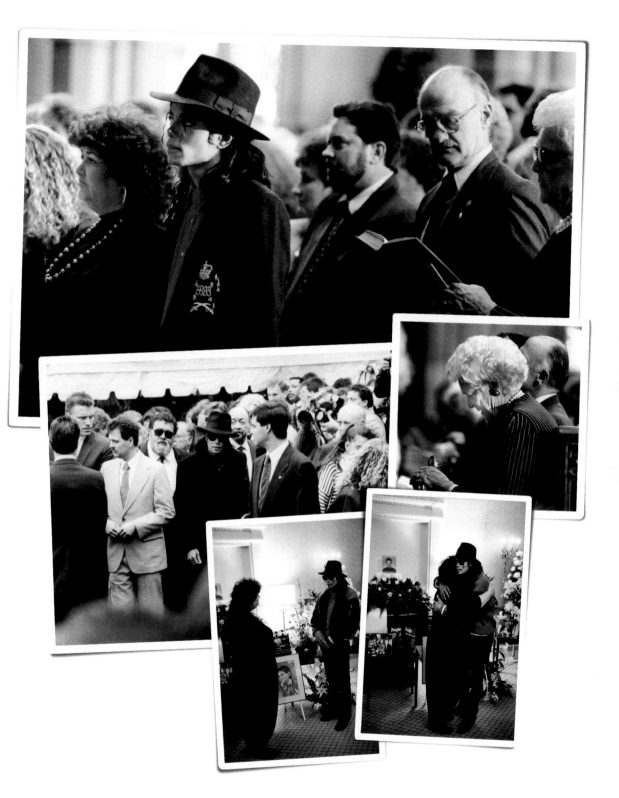

"Well a lot of people will say, 'Your son was such a hero' and all that, but to me, he was my son."

Jeanne White-Ginder

Epilogue

Since Ryan White's death in 1990, major advancements, changes, and developments have occurred. They have impacted everything from the medical treatment of people living with AIDS to the personal lives of Ryan's family members and friends.

A few months after Ryan died, Congress passed, and President George H. W. Bush signed, the Ryan White Care Act. It authorized up to $875 million in funding for programs to help people who tested positive for HIV, the virus that causes AIDS. Nineteen years later, in 2009, President Barack Obama signed the Ryan White HIV/AIDS Treatment Extension Act, the largest federally funded program for people living with HIV in the United States.

Among those invited to the White House when Obama signed the extension was Jeanne White-Ginder. She had gone from being a single mom and factory worker to a crusader who testified before public officials, delivered keynote speeches at conferences, and put together presentations at AIDS awareness events across the country and overseas. "She would get frightened in the beginning, but she's extraordinarily effective in her public speaking," observed Doctor Martin Kleiman, Ryan's physician at Riley Hospital for Children and an infectious disease specialist. "Jeanne has the ability to talk to anyone as if it was a conversation over the backyard

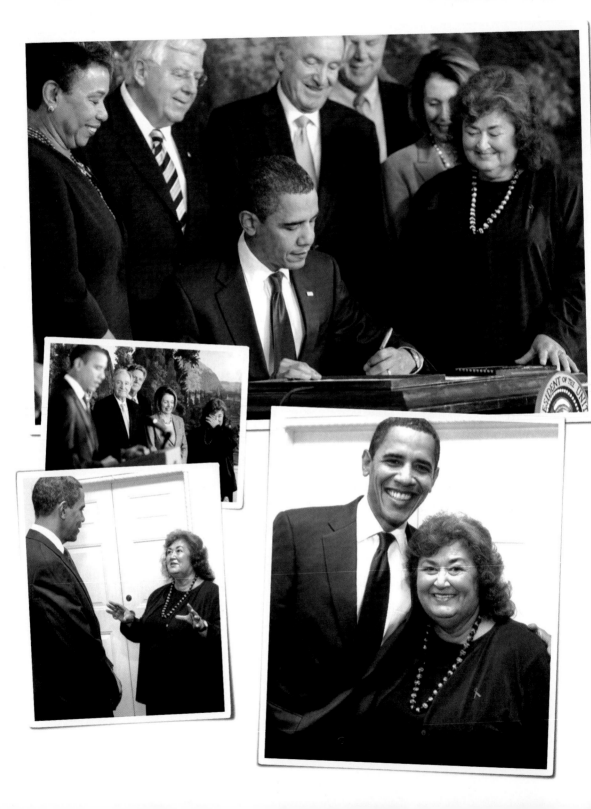

fence. She loved her family, and crusaded for her family. That's what she conveys."

In 1992 Jeanne remarried. She married Roy Ginder, the Cicero neighbor and mechanic who offered to help Ryan customize his beloved Mustang. (Roy also was the single parent who brought his children to the Whites' house on the day of Ryan's death so they could grieve for their friend.)

Although Jeanne met Roy thanks to Ryan, and their shared interest in vintage cars, Ryan's sister Andrea was equally instrumental in the courtship. Alerted about their neighbor's romantic interest in Jeanne, she informed her mother, who hoped to be escorted by a date to a fund-raising event. The date to a fund-raiser led to a courtship.

In the years following her brother's death, Andrea graduated from college and became a sixth-grade teacher in Florida. Jeanne and Roy also have made their home in Florida since the late 1990s.

Jill Stewart, the student body president at Hamilton Heights High School who befriended Ryan, also lives in Florida. Inspired by Kleiman and his interactions with Ryan, Jill decided to pursue a medical career. Doctor Jill Stewart Waibel is a surgeon, wife, and mother in southern Florida.

Ryan's friend, Heather McNew, and his other classmates graduated from Hamilton Heights in 1991, a year after his death. Their yearbook featured a tribute to Ryan written by Heather. She went on to become a special education teacher in Carmel. Heather McNew Stephenson also is a wife and mother. In addition, she became a key organizer of the Special Olympics chapter in Hamilton County.

AIDS remains a worldwide epidemic, but advances in treatment have been dramatic. In the United States, AIDS deaths peaked in 1995, when 50,877 people died across the country. The death rate in America has declined rapidly since then, thanks in large part to highly effective treatments using a variety of medications. Treatment plans usually include combinations of drugs that are specialized for individual patients. The result is that, in the United States, AIDS is regarded as a chronic disorder that can be controlled, not an illness that is inevitably fatal. Still, the impact of AIDS since the early 1980s has been profound, resulting in a total of more than 600,000 deaths in this country by 2012. Also in 2012, about 34.2 million people worldwide were living with HIV. More than 1.1 million of those living with the virus that causes AIDS were Americans. During just 2012 alone, 2.5 million people across the world were infected with HIV.

Since the start of the epidemic in the early 1980s, more than 30 million people have died around the world. Many of the deaths have occurred in African nations where the availability of the latest advancements in medical treatment is extremely limited or nonexistent.

Those advancements in treatment also were not available in April 1990, when Ryan died. His legacy continues in many ways, though. He's been praised by a vast range of Americans—from celebrities to medical workers, teachers, and caregivers—for conveying the need for tolerance toward people struggling with frightening illnesses or with other issues that set them apart from peers. "One of his greatest legacies is increasing the public's understanding of AIDS," said Kleiman, the infectious disease specialist. "He was so special for his young age in his ability to talk directly to kids, to talk to adults, and to talk to the media."

Ryan's accomplishments were honored in Kokomo during an August 2014 tribute that involved a poignant, pubic reconciliation between Jeanne White-Ginder and her hometown. Her son was posthumously inducted into the Howard County Hall of Legends in a ceremony sponsored by the Howard County Historical Society. In accepting the honor for Ryan, Jeanne said she had been skeptical about returning to Kokomo, fearing hostility.

"My husband said to me, 'What would Ryan do?'" she told an audience of nearly 300 people. "I said, 'He'd tell me to go.' " She received a standing ovation when, in remarks that moved some to tears, she summed up her talk this way: "I could not be more proud to be his mother."

As Ryan requested, he is buried in Cicero, his adopted hometown. A small monument marks his gravesite in Cicero Cemetery. "Kid of Courage" is carved into the stone above his birth and death dates. Lyrics from various Elton John songs also are inscribed on the front and back of the monument.

At the base of the monument, a series of descriptive words are inscribed. They include "Faith," "Forgiveness," "Wisdom," and "Tolerance."

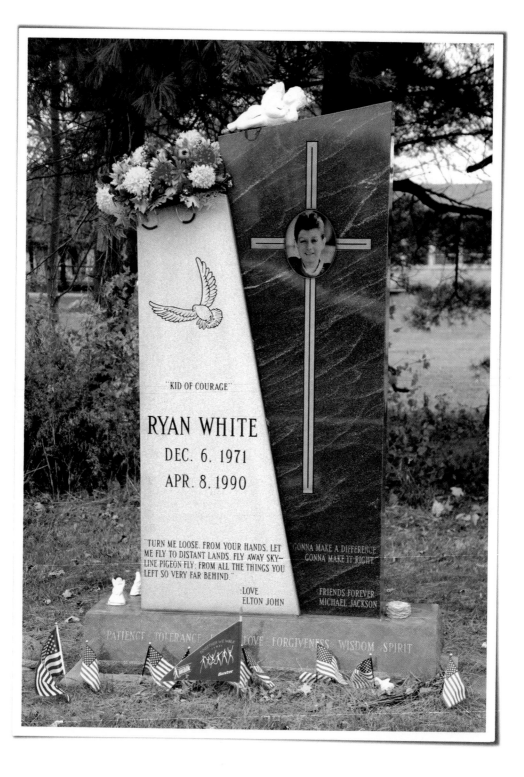

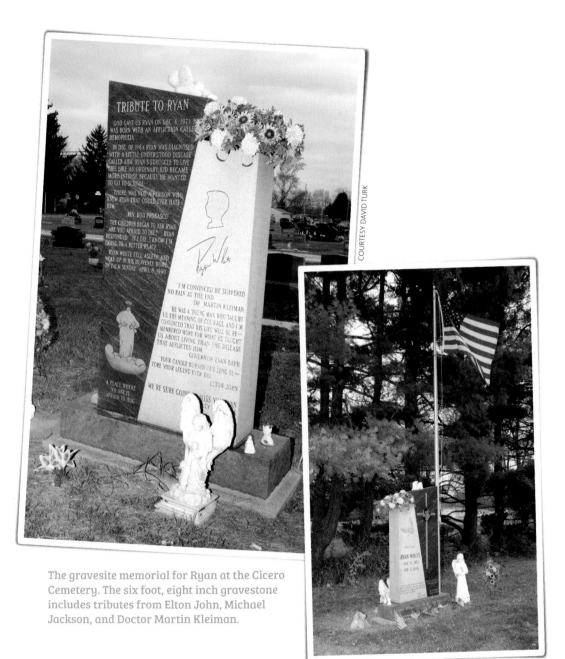

The gravesite memorial for Ryan at the Cicero Cemetery. The six foot, eight inch gravestone includes tributes from Elton John, Michael Jackson, and Doctor Martin Kleiman.

"He was so special for his young age in his ability to talk directly to kids, to talk to adults, and to talk to the media."

Doctor Martin Kleiman

Learn More about Ryan White

Selected Interviews by Nelson Price

Lou Ann Baker, March 31, 2011.

Dan Carter, May 16, 2011.

Ron Colby, June 21, 2011.

Doctor Martin Kleiman, April 8, 2011, and June 18, 2012.

Doctor Woody Myers, March 23, 2011.

Heather McNew Stephenson, March 6, 2011, and May 5, 2012.

Doctor Jill Stewart Waibel, November 16, 2011.

Jeanne White-Ginder, October 22, 2010; October 2, 2011; and July 2, 2012.

Ryan White Oral History Project, Howard County Historical Society, Kokomo, IN

Paula Adair.

Wanda Bowen Bilodeau.

Books

Brill, Marlene Targ. *Extraordinary Young People*. New York: Children's Press, 1996.

Harden, Victoria A. *AIDS at 30: A History*. Dulles, VA: Potomac Books, 2012.

Hoose, Philip M. *We Were There, Too! Young People in U.S. History*. New York: Farrar Straus Giroux, 2001.

John, Elton. *Love Is the Cure: On Life, Loss, and the End of AIDS*. New York: Little, Brown and Company, 2012.

Price, Nelson. *Indiana Legends: Famous Hoosiers from Johnny Appleseed to David Letterman*. Indianapolis: Hawthorne Publishing, 2005.

Resnik, Susan. *Blood Saga: Hemophilia, AIDS, and the Survival of a Community*. Berkeley: University of California Press, 1999.

Shilts, Randy. *And the Band Played On: Politics, People, and the AIDS Epidemic*. Twentieth Anniversary Edition. New York: Saint Martin's Griffin, 2007.

White, Jeanne. *Weeding out the Tears*. With Suzanne Dworkin. New York: Avon Books, 1997.

White, Ryan, and Ann Marie Cunningham. *Ryan White: My Own Story*. New York: Dial Books, 1991.

Magazine/Newspaper Articles

Barrow, Karen. "Changed, but Not Defined, by Hemophilia." *New York Times*, January 31, 2012.

Berry, S. L. "History Experienced through 3 Children's Eyes." *Indianapolis Star*, January 9, 2007.

Bruni, Frank. "The Living after Dying." *New York Times*, March 18, 2012.

Friedman, Jack, and Bill Shaw. "Amazing Grace: The Quiet Victories of Ryan White." *People Magazine*, May 30, 1988.

Johnson, Dick. "Ryan White Dies of AIDS at 18; His Struggle Helped Pierce Myths." *New York Times*, April 9, 1990.

Nichols, Mark. "New Ruling Cuts Short Ryan's School Return." *Indianapolis Star*, February 22, 1986.

Niederpruem, Kyle. "Orr Honors School for Accepting Ryan White." *Indianapolis Star*, December 19, 1987.

Price, Nelson. "Celebrities Cause Stir at White House." *Indianapolis News*, April 9, 1990.

———. "Fame Didn't Change Ryan's Act." *Indianapolis News*, April 9, 1990.

———. "Grandpa Grateful to Ryan." *Indianapolis News*, November 20, 1990.

———."A Quiet Hero: Ryan White Twenty Years Later." *Traces of Indiana and Midwestern History* 22, no. 1 (Winter 2010): 14–23.

———. "Ryan's Mom to Re-wed." *Indianapolis News*, July 21, 1992.

———. "Ryan White: Calling His Own Shots." *Indianapolis News*, April 22, 1986.

———. "Woody Myers in New York." *Indianapolis News*, June 29, 1990.

Reagan, Ronald. "We Owe It to Ryan." *Washington Post*, April 11, 1990.

Safianow, Allen. "Ryan White and Kokomo, Indiana: A City Remembers." *Traces of Indiana and Midwestern History* 25, no. 1 (Winter 2013): 14–25.

Sidewater, Nancy. "The Boy Next Door." *Entertainment Weekly*, April 14, 2000.

Winchell, Susan A. "Discrimination in the Public Schools: Dick and Jane Have AIDS."

William and Mary Law Review 29, no. 4 (1988). http://scholarship.law.wm.edu/wmlr/vol29/iss4/7

Websites

Ryan White Site, http://www.ryanwhite.com/.

Ryan White HIV/AIDS Program, Health Resources and Services Administration HIV/AIDS Programs, U.S. Department of Health and Human Services, http://hab.hrsa.gov /abouthab/aboutprogram.html.

"Who Was Ryan White?" Health Resources and Services Administration HIV/AIDS

Programs, U.S. Department of Health and Human Services, http://hab.hrsa.gov/abouthab /ryanwhite.html.

Index